DR. MICHAEL HUNTER'S

INFLAMMATORY
BREAST CANCER

Hope is being able to see that there is
light despite all of the darkness.

Desmond Tutu

DR. MICHAEL HUNTER'S
INFLAMMATORY BREAST CANCER

PUBLISHED BY CANCERINFO, LLC

Any Internet addresses, phone numbers, or company or product information printed in this book are offered as a resource and are not intended in any way to be or to imply an endorsement by the publisher, nor does the publisher vouch for the existence, content, or services of these sites, phone numbers, companies, or products beyond the life of this book.

 This book is not intended to provide therapy, counseling, or clinical advice or treatment, or to take the place of clinical advice and management from your personal health care provider. Readers are advised to consult their own qualified physicians regarding medical issues. Neither the publisher nor the author take any responsibility for any possible consequences from any treatment, action, or application of information in this book to the reader.

ISBN   9781078186247

Library of Congress Cataloging-in-Publication Data

Names: Hunter, Michael, author.
Title: Dr. Michael Hunter's Inflammatory Breast Cancer / Michael Hunter, M.D.

Identifiers: ISBN 9781078186247

Subjects: LCSHL Breast--Cancer--Epidemiology--Breast--Cancer-Risk factors Breast--Cancer--Management--Inflammatory--Breast--Cancer

Printed in the United States of America

I promised you I would not forget to focus on inflammatory breast cancer.
Fulfilling a promise..

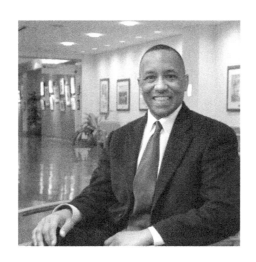

I am a **radiation oncologist** in Seattle (USA), and have degrees from Harvard, Yale, and University of Pennsylvania.

I have served on the Board of Komen Foundation of Puget Sound, as a consultant to the Washington Breast, Cervical, & Colon Health Project, and as cancer program medical director.

Michael Hunter, MD

DR. MICHAEL HUNTER'S

INFLAMMATORY
BREAST CANCER BOOK

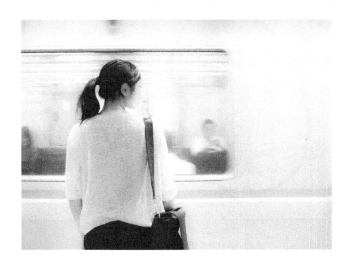

MY MISSION

Inflammatory breast cancer (IBC) is an uncommon and very aggressive disease in which cancer cells block small lymph vessels in the breast skin. This type of breast cancer is called inflammatory because the breast often looks swollen and red, or inflamed.

Surreal. Few words have a greater impact. Some describe the time around hearing "You have breast cancer" as surreal, with some individuals moving from confusion to shock and grief, anger, fear, and despair. If you are experiencing such emotions, you will need time to work through them. Once you do, you should be better able to navigate the journey to becoming more well.

Breast cancer is a story with many chapters. No matter where you find yourself in the journey, I designed this book to help you navigate it. Herein, you will find information about why you may have gotten breast cancer (and basic, sustainable lifestyle adjustments that might improve the odds of it never coming back), what it looks like under the microscope, staging (extent of cancer), prognosis, and cancer management. For brevity, I will not address natural medicine approaches, nor focus on psychological well-being. I hope to be a source of knowledge and support for you.

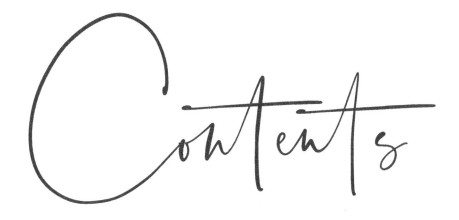

Contents

BASICS

knowledge

INFLAMMATORY BREAST CANCER is an uncommon and rapidly growing form of breast cancer. While other types of breast cancer may form a lump, inflammatory breast cancer spreads along and blocks small lymph vessels in the breast skin. As a result, the lymph vessels become blocked, and the breast becomes red and swollen. This appearance gives inflammatory breast cancer its name.

SYMPTOMS may include:

- a rapid change in breast appearance over weeks
- breast swelling (edema) or lump
- purple or red color of at least one-third of the breast skin
- skin pitting or thickening (orange peel appearance, or peau d'orange)
- unusual breast skin warmth
- enlarged lymph nodes under the arm, or around the collarbone
- the breast may become swollen and enlarged and may feel heavy or uncomfortable
- unusual itchiness

If you have any of these symptoms, it does not necessarily mean that you have inflammatory breast cancer, but you should see a health care provider right away.

13

Inspire

Outcomes improving

Uncommon

Inflammatory breast cancer is uncommon, representing about 2.5 percent of all breast cancers in the United States, but the incidence may be higher elsewhere in the world. In the USA, the incidence appears to be on the rise, especially among white women. By race, the incidence of inflammatory breast cancer is higher among African-Americans, who in turn also tend to be diagnosed at a younger age than their white counterparts.

Hope

Breast cancer death rates in the USA increased by 0.4 percent from 1975 to 1989, but thereafter decreased rapidly (for a total decline of 39 percent through 2015). The decrease occurred among younger and older women, but has slowed among women under 50 since 2007. **This drop in mortality has been associated with improvements in early detection and treatment.**

Not all groups have benefited from these advances equally. A striking divergence in mortality trends among black and white women began in the early 1980s. As management improved, the gap between whites and blacks increased: By 2015, breast cancer death rates were 1.4-times higher among African-American women, compared to their white counterparts.

Inflammatory breast cancer

What about inflammatory breast cancer more specifically? Researchers using the United States Surveillance, Epidemiology and End Results Registry (SEER) identified patients with Stage III (no spread of cancer to distant sites) inflammatory breast cancer diagnosed between 1990 and 2010. They divided patients into four groups, according to year of diagnosis: 1990-1995, 1996-2000, 2001-2005, and 2006-2010.

Researchers found a significant **stepwise improvement in survival over the previous two decades.** The data suggest that improvements in treatment have had a positive impact for women with inflammatory breast cancer.

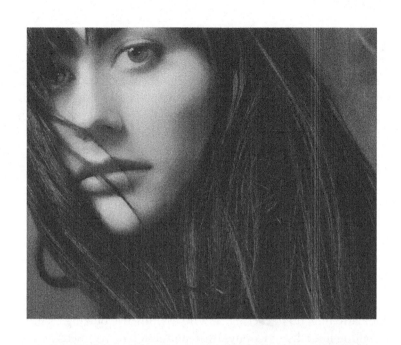

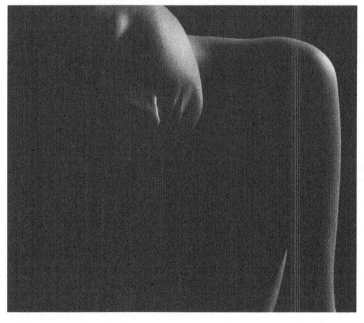

History

Back to the ancient Egyptians

Our oldest description of cancer (although the word cancer was not used) was discovered in Egypt and dates back to 1600 BCE. The Edwin Smith Papyrus is a copy of part of an ancient Egyptian scroll. It describes eight cases of breast tumors or ulcers that were removed by cauterization with a so-called fire drill. The papyrus offered that "there is no treatment." **Sir Charles Bell first described inflammatory breast cancer in 1814.** Still, it was not until 1924 that Lee and Tannebaum (at the suggestion of the pathologist James Ewing) first proposed the use of the term inflammatory breast cancer.

The extent of clinical signs required for inflammatory breast cancer has varied over time. For example, Archibald Leitch in 1909 emphasized the importance of edema, or arm swelling.

> [The breast] is well-modeled from the "artistic point of view" with no flattening, no puckering, and no asymmetric bulging - a diffuse swelling like a hypertrophy. The conjunction of symmetrical hypertrophy and peau d'orange (orange skin) is pathognomic for [defines] inflammatory breast cancer.

He intended the orange skin description to convey an image of minute pits, regularly spaced approximately a quarter of an inch apart, looking as if the breast skin had been dabbed with a blunt pin. Going forward, Haagensen in 1943 emphasized breast redness (erythema), offering that the color may not always be bright red, but rather could have just a "flush of pink." He also observed that the discoloration might (or might not) be uniform, and that it tended to be more prominent in the lower parts of the breast.

French PEV classification

The French PEV (Poussee Evolutive) breast cancer classification system has four components, although only PEV2 and PEV3 would be inflammatory breast cancer in the USA.

> 1. PEV 0: Tumor with no increase in size over the prior 3 months, and no inflammatory signs;
> 2. PEV 1: Tumor with increase in size during the prior 3 months, but with no inflammatory signs.

3. PEV 2: Tumor with associated inflammatory signs (edema/swell-ing, redness,warmth

4. PEV3: Tumor with associated inflammatory signs involving more than half the breast surface

One of the hallmarks of inflammatory breast cancer is the presence of **tumor obstruction of tiny lymphatic vessels in the skin**. This results in the clinical appearance of obstruction. Thomas Bryant described this patho-logic tumor invasion as early as 1887.

Age

In contrast to breast cancer overall, the cancer development process for inflammatory breast cancer is dominated by early-onset types. The age-specific incidence rates increase rapidly until age 50 years old, then flatten or fall for inflammatory breast cancer.

Race

With regard to patient characteristics, patients with inflammatory breast cancer tend to be younger than other breast cancer patients, with a median age at diagnosis of 57 years old for IBC compared to 62 years old for all breast cancers combined. Inflammatory breast cancer has a higher inci-dence rate among black women than white women (3.1 per 100,000 wom-en-years for blacks compared to 2.2 for whites). Further, overall survival has been reported to be significantly worse for blacks than for whites.

Geography

In countries outside the United States, the proportion of breast cancers that are inflammatory breast cancer varies, but is generally higher in the USA.

Menstrual factors

In spite of the fact that inflammatory breast cancer is more commonly found at younger ages than is non-IBC, pre-menopausal status has not consistently been linked with inflammatory breast cancer. Researchers from M.D. Anderson Cancer Center (USA) found 49 percent of IBC cases to be pre-menopausal, compared to 39 percent for non-IBC.

What about age of onset of menstruation, or menarche? It has *not* been consistently associated with inflammatory breast cancer. Researchers at M.D. Anderson Cancer Center (USA) found patients with inflammatory breast cancer to have had a slightly earlier age at menarche, compared to those with non-inflammatory breast cancer cases (12.7 versus 12.2 years of age), but this difference was not statistically significant.

Reproductive factors

Are pregnancy and breast-feeding associated with inflammatory breast cancer risk? Thie clinical literature is mixed, with some studies showing an association and others not.

Body mass index (BMI)

High body mass index is associated with a decreased risk for breast cancer among pre-menopausal (but not post-menopausal women). Does the same link hold true for inflammatory breast cancer? M.D. Anderson Cancer Center (USA) researchers studied women with inflammatory breast cancer diagnosed between 1985 and 1996. They pair-matched 68 patients with inflammatory breast cancer with 143 patients with non-IBC and 134 with no history of breast cancer, according to date of diagnosis and race. Here's what they found:

> **The highest body mass index (BMI over 26.65 kilograms per meter squared) was associated with an increased risk for inflammatory breast cancer,** compared to non-inflammatory breast cancer. This risk increased by a factor of 2.45, and the relationship held true when controlling for menopausal status, age at menopause, family history of breast cancer, number of pregnancies, smoking status, and alcohol use.

Smoking, alcohol, and family history

These researchers found former (and current) users of cigarettes have a *lower* risk of inflammatory breast cancer, compared to non-smokers. There does not appear to be an association between IBC and alcohol use. Finally, while thirteen percent of those with inflammatory breast cancer had a family history of breast cancer (higher than the eight percent found among those with non-inflammatory breast cancer), the difference was not statistically significant.

Males

Like other types of breast cancer, inflammatory breast cancer can occur in men, but usually at an older age than in women.

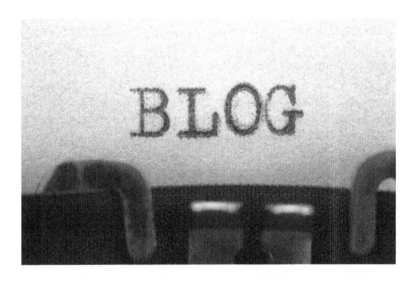

www.newcancerinfo.com

Diet: Breast cancer in general

Diet

A Mediterranean diet (rich with plant foods, fish and olive oil) is associated with better heart health. A Spanish study suggests it *may* also reduce the risk of developing breast cancer. Investigators randomly assigned more than 4,200 women, ages 60 to 80, to eat either a Mediterranean diet supplemented with extra virgin olive oil or with nuts, versus a low-fat control diet. The women, who joined the study in 2003 to 2009 were all at high risk for heart disease, and their average body mass index was 30 (considered obese; obesity is itself a risk factor for the development of post-menopausal breast cancer). Less than 3 percent had used hormone therapy, and the average age was 68.

Compared with the control diet group, the **Mediterranean plus olive oil group had a 68 percent lower risk of developing breast cancer** over a five year follow-up period. While the Mediterranean diet with nuts reduced risk, the results were not statistically significant. There are some limitations to the study, including the fact that breast cancer was *not* the primary subject of the research. In addition, it is unclear whether the olive oil was beneficial on its own, or only when taken with the Mediterranean diet.

How much olive oil?

Women in the study consumed four tablespoons daily, using it as a spread, for salads, and for cooking. Those in the nut consumption group ate about an ounce of nuts daily, half walnuts and the other half split between hazelnuts and almonds. While the results seem promising, we need longer follow-up, and validation studies. Still, this PREDIMED study adds to growing support for the health benefits of a Mediterranean-type diet.

A systematic review also suggests the Mediterranean dietary pattern (and diets composed largely of vegetables, fruit, fish, and soy) is associated with a decreased risk of breast cancer. Researchers found no association between traditional dietary patterns and the risk of getting breast cancer, and only one study showed a significant increase in risk associated with the Western dietary pattern. For those who already have breast cancer, I am unaware of an effect of any particular diet on prognosis, but generally suggest adherence to a balanced diet, including copious fruits and vegetables (and not much red meat).

Modifiable: Blue light at night

Exposure to light

Light at night is bad for your health, and exposure to blue light emitted by electronics and energy-efficient lightbulbs may be especially so. Here is an excerpt from the *Harvard Health Letter:*

> "Until the advent of artificial lighting, the sun was the major source of lighting, and people spent their evenings in (relative) darkness. Now, in much of the world, evenings are illuminated, and we take our easy access to all those lumens for granted. But we may be paying a price for basking in all that light. At night, light throws the body's biological clock—the circadian rhythm—out of whack. Sleep suffers. Worse, research shows that it may contribute to the causation of cancer, diabetes, heart disease, and obesity."

Night shift

Many (but certainly not all) studies have linked working night shift to a higher risk of breast and prostate cancer, diabetes, heart disease, and obesity. It's not entirely clear why night time light exposure seems to be so bad for us. We do know that exposure to light drops your melatonin, a hormone that influences our awake/sleep rhythms. There is some limited evidence that lower melatonin levels might explain the association with cancer.

Type of light: The blues

Melatonin is a hormone in your body that plays a role in sleep. The production and release of melatonin in the brain is connected to time of day, increasing when it's dark and decreasing when it's light. Melatonin production declines with age. While light of any color can suppress melatonin, blue light/wavelengths (beneficial during daylight hours because they boost attention, reaction times, and mood) seem to be the most disruptive at night. Exposure to electronics with screens (and energy-efficient lighting) is increasing our exposure to blue wavelengths, especially after sundown. Harvard researchers examined the effects of 6.5 hours of blue light exposure with exposure to green light of comparable brightness. The blue light suppressed melatonin for about twice as long as the green light and shifted the natural 24 hour cycle by twice as much (3 hours vs. 1.5 hours).

Changeable: Lifestyle

Physical Activity

Physical activity may lower the risk of breast cancer, especially for women who have gone through menopause. Exercise can lower estrogen levels, fight obesity and boost immune system cells that attack tumors.

• Before you start an exercise program, please consult a valued health care provider. This is especially important if you have been inactive for a long time, are overweight, have a high risk of heart disease, or have a high risk of other chronic health problems.

• **Include physical activity in your daily routine.** Aim for the minimum of the equivalent of a brisk walk for 30 minutes daily.

Weight

• Gaining weight after menopause increases breast cancer risk.

• Weight gain of 20 pounds or more after the age of 18 *may* increase your risk of breast cancer.

• If you have gained weight, losing weight may lower your risk of breast cancer. **Aim for a body mass index (BMI) of 20 to 25.**

Breastfeeding

Breastfeeding can *lower* risk.

Alcohol

Having one serving of alcohol (for example, a glass of red wine) each day *may* improve your health by reducing your risk of heart disease and stroke. However, alcohol can increase your breast cancer risk: The more you drink, the higher the risk. If you drink alcohol, certainly aim for less than one standard drink a day, on average. Getting enough folic acid *may* lower the risk linked to drinking alcohol, but the evidence here is not high-level. You can find folic acid in multivitamins, oranges, orange juice, green vegetables and fortified breakfast cereals.

RISKS (breast cancer in general)

	Lower	Higher	RR*
BRCA mutation	Negative	Positive	3 to 7x increase
Mother or sister with breast cancer	No	Yes	2.6
Age	30 to 34	70 to 74	18
Age at menarche	Over 14	Less than 12	1.5
Age at first birth	Under 20	Over 30	1.9 to 3.5
Age at menopause	Under 45	Over 55	2
Use of contraceptive pills	Never	Past/current	1.1 to 1.2
Estrogen + progestin	Never	Current	1.2
Alcohol	None	2 to 5/day	1.4
Breast density	0	75 or higher	1.8 to 6
Bone density	Lowest quartile	Highest quartile	2.7 to 3.5
History of benign breast biopsy	No	Yes	1.7
History of atypical hyperplasia	No	Yes	3.7

Protective

Breastfeeding (months)	16 or more	0	0.7
Full-term pregnancies	5 or more	0	0.7
Exercise	Yes	No	0.7
Postmenopausal BMI	Under 22.9	Over 30.7	0.6
Ovaries removed before age 35	Yes	No	0.3
Aspirin	More than once per week, 6+ months	Non-user	0.8

* relative risk

Triple negative

Triple negative breast cancer (TNBC) is a term that we often apply to cancers that are low in expression of estrogen receptors (ER) and progesterone receptors (PR), as well as human epidermal factor receptor 2 (HER2). TNBC often behaves more aggressively than other breast cancer types. Triple negative breast cancer accounts for about 20 percent of breast cancers worldwide, and is more commonly diagnosed among women younger than 40 years compared with estrogen- or progesterone-receptor positive breast cancer. In fact the risk of TNBC is about doubled among those under 40, as compared with women over 50. Let's look at some ot the risks unique to triple negative breast cancer:

Breast cancer genes, inherited

Up to 20 percent of patients with triple negative breast cancer have a breast cancer gene (BRCA) mutation, more common with BRCA1 (than BRCA2). By contrast, less than 6 percent of all breast cancers are linked to BRCA. In general, if you have TNBC and are 60 years or younger, you should have genetic testing.

Race

African-Americans have a significantly higher risk of triple negative breast cancer, as compared to non-African-American women.

Pre-menopausal

Pre-menopausal status has been associated with TNBC.

Maternal

Breast-feeding may lower risk, at least according to some (but not all) studies. As well, limited data suggests that younger age at first pregnancy may *increase* the risk of TNBC. Finally, those who have had no full-term pregnancies may have a higher risk; on the other hand, there are hints that having three or more births may *increase* the risk of TNBC, but there is not compelling evidence.

Other hormonal factors

Some (but not all) studies have linked other hormonal factors (early age to start menstruating; ongoing hormone replacement therapy; oral contraceptive use) to triple negative breast cancer.

TRIPLE NEGATIVE BREAST CANCER (TNBC)

The most common receptors known to fuel most breast cancer growth – estrogen, progesterone, and HER-2 receptors– are not present in the cancer cells.

Male breast cancer

Risk factors

Here is some information about breast cancer overall, **not specific to the inflammatory type.** Aging is a significant risk factor for male breast cancer. The risk of breast cancer increases with age with an average age at diagnosis of 68.

Family history; genes

Breast cancer risk increases if blood relatives have had breast cancer. About one in five men with breast cancer have a close male or female relative with the disease. Men with a mutation (defect) in the BRCA2 gene (BReast CAncer gene 2) have an elevated lifetime risk of about 6 in 100. BRCA1 mutations also raise breast cancer risk to about 1 in 100. Although gene mutations are most often found in members of families with many cases of breast and/or ovarian cancer, they can occur in men with breast cancer who do not have a strong family history. Mutations in CHEK2 and PTEN genes also raise risk.

Klinefelter syndrome

Klinefelter syndrome is a congenital (present at birth) condition that affects one in 1000 men. Normally the cells in mens' bodies have a single X chromosome along with a Y chromosome, while womens' cells have two X chromosomes. Men with Klinefelter syndrome have cells with a Y chromosome plus at least two X chromosomes (and sometimes more). These men typically have smaller than normal testicles, and many cannot produce functioning sperm and are therefore infertile. Compared with other men, they have lower levels of male hormones (androgens) and more estrogens ("female" hormones). Given this, many develop gynecomastia (non-cancer male breast growth).

Some studies have found that men with Klinefelter syndrome are more likely to get breast cancer: One study reported a breast cancer risk of one in 100. Estimating risk is tough, as the numbers of individuals with the condition are small. The risk may be higher, but overall it is still low because this is such an uncommon cancer, even among men with Klinefelter syndrome.

Estrogen

Estrogen-related drugs were once used as hormonal therapy for men with prostate cancer. Estrogen may slightly increase breast cancer risk. Transgender/transsexual individuals who take high doses of estrogens as part of a sex reassignment may also have a higher breast cancer risk. As we don't have any studies of breast cancer risk among transgendered individuals, the actual breast cancer risk is unclear.

Alcohol

Heavy consumption of alcohol-containing beverages increases breast cancer risk among men. This may be because of its effects on the liver. The liver binds proteins that carry hormones in the blood, proteins that affect hormone activity. Men with severe liver diseases such as cirrhosis have relatively low levels of male hormones and higher estrogen levels. They have a higher rate of benign male breast growth (gynecomastia), and a higher risk of developing breast cancer.

Obesity

Obesity is a likely risk factor for male breast cancer. Fat cells convert so-called male hormones (androgens) into "female" hormones (estrogens). Obese men have higher levels of estrogens in their body.

Testicular conditions

Certain conditions, such as having an undescended testicle, having mumps as an adult, or having one or both testicles surgically removed may increase male breast cancer risk. Although the risk appears to be increased, it is low.

Certain occupations

There may be an increased risk among men who work in very hot environments such as steel mills. Exposure to higher temperatures for long periods can affect the testicles, which can then affect hormone levels. Men heavily exposed to gasoline fumes may also have a higher risk.

While male breast cancer has been on a slow rise since 1975, **male breast cancer death rates have dropped** by about 1.8 percent per year since 2000.

Breast cancer risk

Calculators

Risk assessments are designed to educate patients about cancer risk, determine if genetic testing is indicated, and help decide when breast cancer screening with mammograms should start. High-risk patients can be offered screening breast magnetic resonance imaging (MRI) in addition to annual mammograms and chemoprevention to help reduce breast cancer risk,

Various risk-prediction models have been created for breast cancer. We may conveniently stratify women into one of three risk groups for the development of breast cancer:

> • **Average risk (75% of women):** No family history of the disease and no significant personal risk factors (for example, a previous biopsy of the breast) that would constitute a higher risk. Those in the average risk group have a 12% chance of developing breast cancer.

> • **Women with hereditary breast cancer** risk and a genetic mutation known to confer a high lifetime risk (12% of women).

> • **Moderate risk:** Women with a family history of breast cancer not associated with known genes, or women who have had a breast biopsy that shows a precancerous change.

There are several credible online tools available to help women and their care providers better understand breast cancer risk. Such knowledge may help inform your decision-making regarding breast cancer risk reduction strategies, genetic counseling/testing options, and screening options for the earlier detection of breast cancer. Alas, there is no tool that can predict with certainty your individual risk, and each test has both strengths and limitations. Let's look at some of these tools.

Risk assessment tool for the general public

Your Disease Risk *(www.yourdiseaserisk.wustl.edu)* is a wonderful website from Washington University (USA) that offers both educational material and a risk assessment tool for breast cancer (and other diseases as well). It puts you into above average, average, or below average risk categories, compared to the general population. I really like this relatively easy to use tool. The tool was developed using data for the USA, and estimates your risk relative to the US general population. In addition, the tool only considers limited information about your family history of breast cancer, which could lead to underestimating risk for some patients.

Risk assessment tools for health professionals

Many of these tools are accessible to you online. Still, if you choose to explore any of them, please discuss your results with a valued health care provider.

What	Factors	Notes
Gail model	Previous breast biopsies (and whether atypia is present); reproductive history (age at start of menstruation and age at first live birth of a child); family history of breast cancer among first-degree relatives (e.g. mother; sister; daughter)	• Only considers limited info about family breast cancer history • Does not include factors such as use of hormone replacement therapy, breast density, and lifestyle factors such as smoking, alcohol use, diet, or physical inactivity
Breast Cancer Risk Assessment Tool	Age; age at first menarche; age at first live birth of a child; family and personal history of breast cancer;	• A 5-year risk of 1.67% or higher is considered high risk for developing breast cancer
IBIS (Tyrer-Cuzick) Breast Cancer Risk Evaluation Tool	Age; age at first live birth of a child; age at first period; age at menopause; height and weight; prior risk-increasing benign biopsy of breast; use of hormones; comprehensive family history	• Does not include risk factors associated with lifestyle or breast density • Genetic counseling advised when the model predicts a 10% or higher chance that you have a mutation of BRCA

At high risk?

Risk-reducing bilateral mastectomy

Today, many high-risk women are choosing to have surgical removal of both breasts as a means of reducing their risk of developing breast cancer in the future. While such a radical move reduces risk, it remains unclear as to whether it has a significant impact on survival odds. Still, some women at high risk choose removal of both breasts as they feel the complications associated with the surgery are worth the benefits (psychological; desire for symmetry; reduced need for future mammogram surveillance).

The primary goal of bilateral prophylactic (risk-reducing) mastectomy is to reduce breast cancer risk. Here are estimated risks, based on various factors:

Genetic risk factors	Lifetime risk
BRCA1	81%
BRCA2	85%
p53	24%
PTEN	25%

Non-genetic risk factors	Relative risk
Classic LIN*	7 to 11x
ADH/ALH*	4 to 5x
Proliferative change, without atypia	1.9x

* LIN lobular intraepithelial neoplasia
 ADH atypical ductal hyperplasia
 ALH atypical lobular hyperplasia

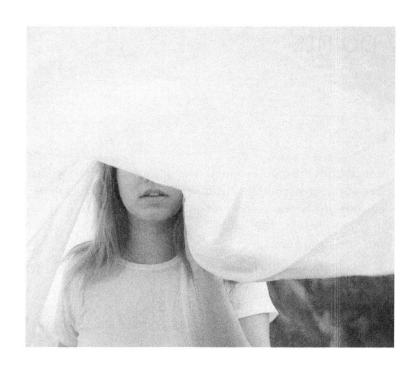

High risk? Consider:

	Relative risk drop
Tamoxifen (pills)	37-49%
Raloxifene (pills)	56-59%
Exemestane (pills)	65%
Removal of both ovaries	53%
Removal of both breasts	90-100%

Key points

Risk

Breast cancer remains the most common non-skin cancer among women in the United States. Fortunately, mortality from breast cancer continues to decline. We may conveniently divide risk factors into one of three major groups:

- Inherited genetics
- Hormone-related (including reproductive factors)
- Environmental

Inflammatory breast cancer risk factors include obesity and female sex. African-American women appear to have a higher risk, too.

Action list

Many risk factors are not easily modifiable. Still, let's focus on the ones that are potentially changeable:

- **Physical activity:** Aim for the equivalent of a brisk walk for 150 minutes per week (for example, 30 minutes for 5 days per week).

- **Weight:** Shoot for a Body Mass Index (BMI) of 20 to 25.

- **Alcohol:** Be prudent, limiting consumption to no more than 3 to 7 standard drinks per week (and not more than 3 at any given time).

- **Diet:** Preferred diets include ones that are relatively low in fat, and rich in fruits and vegetables. Incorporate extra virgin olive oil into your diet, perhaps as much as four tablespoons per day!

- **Anti-estrogen (endocrine) therapy:** If you are on these pills, don't forget to take them as prescribed.

- **Hormones:** Combined long-term use of estrogen and progestin menopausal hormone replacement therapy *increases* breast cancer risk.

courage

IMAGE

Clinical features

Inflammatory breast cancer

Individuals with inflammatory breast cancer (IBC) typically present with:

- breast discomfort
- a rapidly growing, self-diagnosed mass
- a firm, tender, or enlarged breast
- itchiness of a breast
- redness of the breast

Rapid onset

The onset of IBC symptoms is usually very rapid, often over weeks to months. Many will be treated with antibiotics first, under the presumption that the symptoms are due to breast infection, or mastitis.

Cancer spread

Unfortunately, virtually all patients with inflammatory breast cancer will have spread to regional lymph nodes (for example, in the underarm/axillary region). In this context, some women may report swelling of their underarm lymph nodes, or discomfort in that area. At diagnosis, about one-third of patients will have distant spread (metastases) to organs such as the bones, liver, lung, or brain.

Physical exam

Typical signs of the affected breast may include:

- Skin warmth
- Skin thickening
- Orange peel appearance (peau d'orange) of skin
- Discoloration (range from pink to red or purplish hue)
- Nipple changes (flattening, redness, crusting, blisters, or retraction)
- Breast mass that can be felt

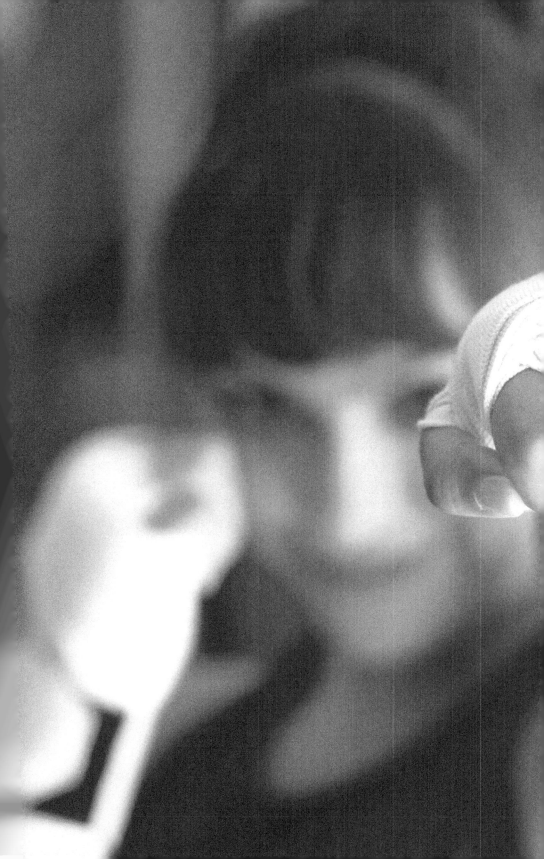

Tools

mam•mo•gram Images of the breast, obtained using X-rays.

Mammograms are the foundation of screening for women
at average risk of getting the disease. Several randomized trials comparing screening mammograms versus no screening
mammograms have shown that this imaging test decreases the
odds of dying from breast cancer. Digital mammograms and
tomosynthesis (3D mammograms) are more recent innovations.
**Screening mammograms trigger the diagnosis of inflamma-
tory breast cancer in less than ten percent of cases.**

ul•tra•sound Images of the breast, obtained using sound waves.

Ultrasound is commonly used as a diagnostic follow-up when
there is something concerning on mammograms. While not
generally used as a screening tool for women at average risk,
some centers will incorporate ultrasound into screening for
highly select women with increased breast density.

MRI Images of the breast, obtained using powerful magnets.

Magnetic resonance imaging (MRI) is used for breast cancer
diagnosis and staging. In addition, MRI may be used as a screening tool for women at higher risk, or to assess response to chemotherapy. Breast MRI uses magnetic fields and an intravenous (IV)
contrast agent to create images of the breast.

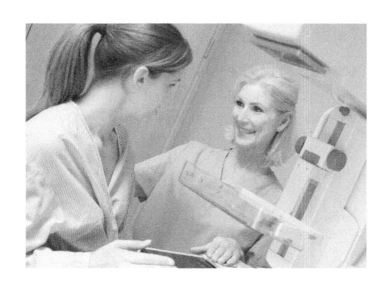

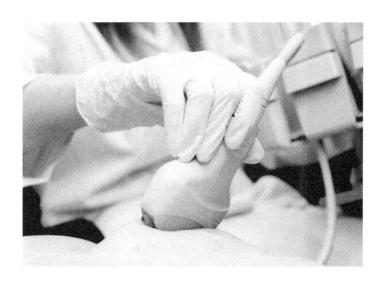

Mammograms

to·mo·SYN·the·sis

Tomosynthesis is a form of digital mammograms that creates a **3-D** picture of the breast using X-rays.

What

A regular mammogram typically takes two X-rays of each breast (one from top to bottom, and the other side to side). Digital tomosynthesis takes multiple X-ray pictures of each breast from many angles. The breast is positioned in a way similar to standard mammograms, but less pressure is applied.

The X-ray tube moves in an arc around the breast while multiple images are taken over about seven seconds. The information is then sent to a computer, where it is assembled to create clear 3D images of the breast. These multiple pictures create a layer-by-layer look at the breast tissue — one millimeter at a time — removing tissue overlap that may hide cancers or mistake dense breast tissue for cancer.

Why

Results with tomosynthesis are quite promising. Tomosynthesis can make breast cancers easier to see, especially in dense breast tissue, and may reduce the chances you will be called back for additional studies.

Better detection, fewer recalls

In one large study, researchers looked at data from 13 medical centers before and after they began using tomosynthesis. Digital mammograms with tomosynthesis detected one additional cancer for every 1,000 scans and resulted in 15% fewer false alarms – women called back for more tests and then found not to have cancer. The study was not designed to find out whether mammograms using tomosynthesis can save more lives than standard digital mammograms.

The bottom line? Investigators found that the use of tomosynthesis ("3D") mammograms was associated with:

- Improved cancer detection rates, especially invasive cancers

- A decrease in call backs, which may lessen anxiety for patients

No access to tomosynthesis?

Dr. Robert Smith, American Cancer Society senior director of cancer screening, offers that the study described above does not mean all women should seek out 3-D mammograms. Although the study showed an important improvement in cancer detection rates, the improvement was small. The more dramatic finding, he observes, was having a lower chance of being called back for additional testing; that is, as compared to standard mammograms, tomosynthesis resulted in fewer false positives.

Step into the forest...

I love this analogy from *www.breastcancer.org:* Traditional mammograms take only one picture, across the entire breast, in two directions: Top to bottom and side to side. It's like standing on the edge of a forest, looking for a bird somewhere inside. To find the bird, it would be better to take 10 steps at a time through the forest and look all around you with each move. Welcome to the world of the 3-D mammogram, tomosynthesis. A radiologist analyzes the results of your exam and sends a report to your personal physician. For non-emergency situations, it usually takes a day or so to interpret, report, and deliver the results.

Did you know...

The Food and Drug Administration (FDA) approved breast tomosynthesis for use in February, 2011. By the following month, the Harvard Massachusettes General Hospital breast imaging team performed the first clinical breast tomosynthesis exam in the United States.

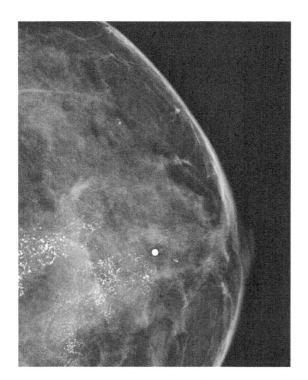

Mammogram
Malignant (cancer) calcifications

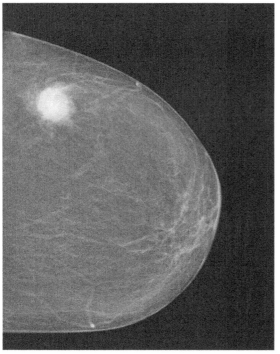

Mammogram
Mass (cancer)

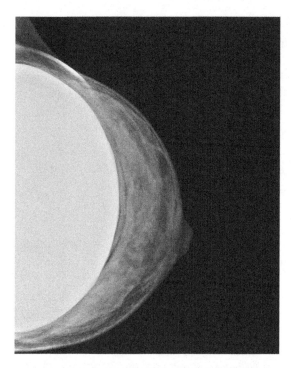

Mammogram
Implant obscures
tissue

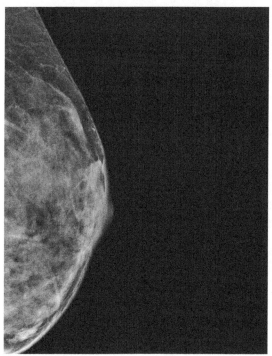

Mammogram
Cancer calcifications
Implant displacement
(pushed away) view

If you have an abnormal mammogram or a concerning physical finding, what's next? Follow-up typically begins with less invasive tests such as
diagnostic mammograms or breast ultrasound. The radiologist examines
the images to determine whether the abnormal finding looks suspicious:

• *Not suspicious-appearing*

If the lesion clearly doesn't look like cancer on imaging, you may not need
any more testing. An example is a simple cyst.

• *Suspicious-appearing*

Typically, a biopsy (a tissue sampling, often using a needle) is done, and
the abnormal tissue then sent to a pathologist to examine it for cancer.

Most calcifications seen on mammograms are *not* cancer. However, calcifications are sometimes a sign of cancer. We may conveniently classify calcifications into one of 3 categories:

1) Benign
2) Intermediate concern
3) Higher probability of cancer

Benign calcifications are typically larger, coarser, and round with smooth margins. They may be scattered or diffuse. Malignant calcifications are typically
grouped or clustered, pleomorphic (varying in size and shape), fine and with
linear branching.

Mammogram: Screening versus Diagnostic

Screening mammograms are used for individuals with no symptoms or signs
of breast cancer. Screening mammograms try to find breast cancer when it is
too small to be felt by you or your care provider. Diagnostic mammograms are
used for individuals with a known breast problem. Examples include a lump or
nipple discharge, or an abnormal area found in a screening mammogram. We
sometimes use diagnostic mammograms for patients without breast problems
who were previously treated for breast cancer. During a diagnostic mammogram, the images are reviewed by the radiologist while you are there, so that
more images may be obtained if needed to look at a concerning area.

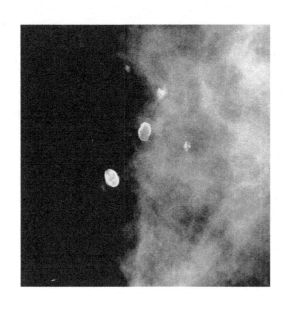

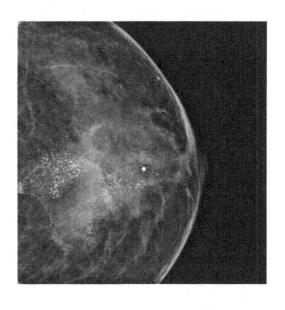

Diagnostic mammograms

Sometimes, special images known as spot (or magnification) views are taken, in order to make a small area of concern easier to evaluate. Diagnostic mammograms may be interpreted in one of 3 ways:

> • **Not cancer:** An area that looked abnormal on a screening mammogram appears normal. You typically then return to routine annual mammograms.

> • **Probably not cancer:** An area that looked abnormal on a screening mammogram is probably not cancer, but it is common to be asked to come back in 4 to 6 months to re-check.

> • **Looks like may be cancer:** A biopsy is recommended.

A photograph of the breast at presentation may be useful in monitoring changes over time.

Special case: Women under 30 with symptoms

For women under 30, most breast lumps are benign (not cancer). A first step is a clinical breast exam (CBE), a physical exam performed by a skilled health care provider. The clinician should carefully feel your breasts and underarm area for any changes abnormalities (such as a lump). Examples of abnormal findings that may be discovered on clinical exam include:

- A dominant lump in the breast or underarm area
- Change in breast size or shape
- Dimpling or puckering of skin
- Pulling in of the nipple or other breast parts
- Nipple discharge
- Pain
- Swelling, redness, warmth, or darkening of the breast

Additional evaluation may include a breast ultrasound (and for selected women, a mammogram). Selected women may require a biopsy to determine whether a lump is breast cancer or not.

MAMMOGRAMS

BI-RADS Category*	
1 Negative	No significant abnormality.
2 Benign	No sign of cancer, but the reporting radiologist chooses to describe a finding thought benign (e.g. benign calcifications).
3 Probably benign	98% chance *not* cancer. May be suggested to repeat imaging in 6 months, and regularly thereafter to ensure stability.
4 Suspicious	Findings do not definitely look like cancer, but could be. Radiologist concerned enough to recommend a biopsy.
5 Highly suggestive of cancer	High chance (over 95%) cancer present. Biopsy is strongly recommended.
6 Known cancer	May be used to assess reponse to treatment.

* We use a standard system to describe mammogram findings and results. This system (called the Breast Imaging Reporting and Data System or BI-RADS) sorts results into categories as above. By categorizing in this way, we can describe the mammogram findings using the common terminology. This makes accurately communicating about test results (and recommended) much easier.

Breast density

Breast density may be reported on your mammogram report, but is often sub-jective. In addition to a BI-RADS system describing our level of suspicion (see table to the right), the BI-RADS system also classifies breast density:

> • *Almost entirely fatty*
> Because fatty breasts have little fibrous and glandular tissue, the mammogram would likely be able to see anything abnormal.

> • *Having scattered fibroglandular density*
> There are a few areas of fibrous and glandular tissue in the breast.

> • *Heterogeneously dense*
> The breast has more areas of fibrous and glandular tissue throughout the breast. This can make finding small masses more challenging.

> • *Extremely dense*
> The breast has a lot of fibrous and glandular tissue. This can make it harder to see a cancer, as it can blend in with normal tissues (like finding a snowball in a snow field).

Dense breasts have a significantly higher risk of developing breast cancer. But does the presence of dense breasts among those with breast cancer af-fect the risk of dying of the disease? To examine the relationship between breast density and breast cancer mortality, researchers analyzed data from the Breast Cancer Surveillance Consortium (BCSC), a population-based registry of breast imaging facilities in the USA. They limited data collec-tion to the five BCSC registries that consistently collect data on body mass index (BMI), in order to be able to adjust for such factors.

After adjusting for other health factors, the analysis showed that the overall group of patients with high-density breasts did not have a higher risk of death from breast cancer, as compared with patients with lower density breasts. However, subgroup analysis suggested that there might be an increased risk of breast cancer death among women with low density (BI-RADS 1) who were either obese (2-times increase in risk) or had primary cancers measuring 2cm or greater (1.55-times increase in risk).

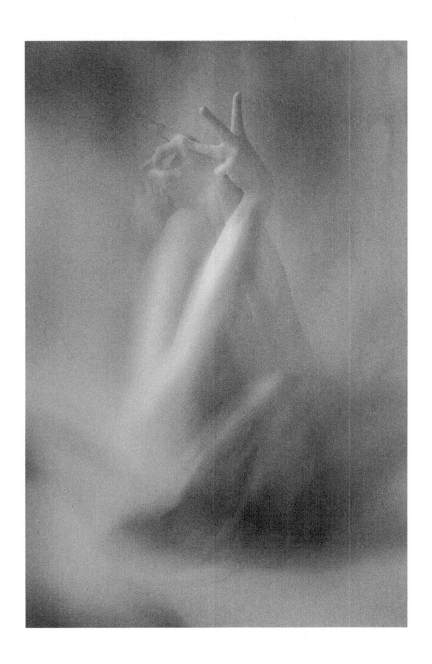

3
BIOPSY

Biopsy types

Removal of cells or tissue from the breast skin and/or breast itself for examination under a microscope is known as a biopsy. This may be done under local anaesthetic. If any axillary (underarm) nodes seem enlarged, a biopsy of a lymph node may be performed.

Least invasive

A needle biopsy uses a hollow needle to remove samples of tissue or cells from the breast. The material is then sent to a pathologist, who studies these samples under a microscope to see if they contain cancer or other concerning findings.

- **Core needle biopsy; punch biopsy**

   These are the preferred ways to make the initial diagnosis of inflammatory breast cancer. Core needle biopsy removes a narrow cylinder of tissue. While there is a small chance of bruising or infection, it is generally accurate, and (if a cancer is present) can provide information about the cancer type, grade (aggressiveness), and receptor status (Is the cancer driven by estrogen? Progesterone? HER2?). **A full thickness skin punch biopsy** (preferably two) is often performed. The pathologist can then look for invasion of the small lymphatic channels by cancer, a phenomenon usually present with inflammatory breast cancer.

- **Fine needle aspiration (FNA)**

   A core and/or punch biopsy is preferred. FNA removes cells from a suspicious lump, and is only used for lumps that can be felt. The needle used is thinner than ones used for core needle biopsies. While core needle biopsy is often the first choice for palpable masses, FNA is sometimes done as a quick means of sampling a breast lump felt during a clinical breast exam or a concerning underarm (axillary) lymph node. The false positive rate is about 1 to 2%. The false negative rate (the cancer is present, but the biopsy doesn't show it) can be on the order of 40%, so if the FNA does not show cancer, your care team will recommend the obtaining of more tissue.

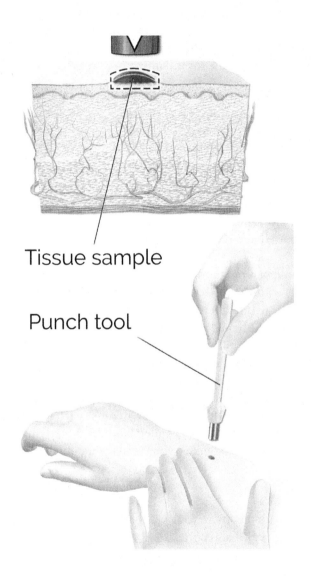

Tissue sample

Punch tool

Excisional biopsy (continued)

The incision should be long enough to provide adequate exposure and to ensure that the mass can be removed as a single specimen with a small margin of grossly normal tissue. The surgeon should orient the specimen, and the pathologist should ink all margins. Excisional biopsy is not typically done for inflammatory breast cancer.

Results

After tissue is removed, the material is sent to a doctor known as a **pathologist.** The pathologist examines the tissue, including with the use of a microscope and determines whether the tissue contains cancer. A pathology report (including the diagnosis) is issued, and sent to the ordering physician. The report may have material added at a later date, so there can be more than one report for a single biopsy session.

Your pathology report provides your diagnosis. Most of the initial information comes within 7 to 10 days after your surgery, and you will usually have all the results within a few weeks. Your doctor can let you know when the results come in. If you don't hear from your doctor, call the office. A physician (such as your radiologist, surgeon or oncologist) will review the main findings of the report and answer any questions you may have. The report itself is prepared for healthcare providers, making the language sometimes confusing for the patient. Still, understanding the basic parts of the report can help you to be a better consumer. Because each individual's breast cancer is unique, it's important to understand the underlying biology of your cancer in order to personalize your management plan.

 Ask for a copy of your pathology report (and other test results) for your personal records.

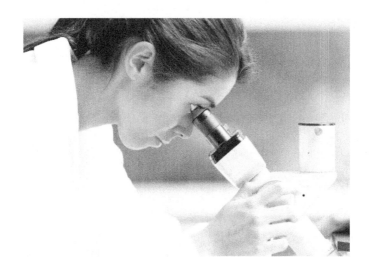

1 **Pathologist** receives biopsy material.

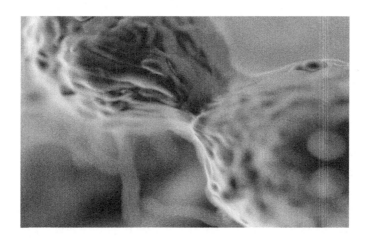

2 Tissue examined under a microscope.

Basics

Cancer is a condition in which cells do not die at the normal rate. As the cell growth exceeds cell death, a mass of tissue (tumor) can form. Breast cancer happens when cells in the breast divide and grow abnormally. Up to 75% of breast cancers begin in the milk ducts, while 10 to 15% begin in the lobules. The remainder start in other breast tissues. **Benign** means not cancer.

Non-invasive or invasive?

We may conveniently divide breast cancer into two categories: Invasive versus non-invasive breast cancer. The latter is also referred to as ductal carcinoma *in situ* (DUK-tul kar-sin-O-ma in SY-too), or DCIS. Only about 20 to 25% of breast cancer is non-invasive. **Inflammatory breast cancer is invasive.**

> • Ductal carcinoma *in situ* (DCIS)
> Abnormal cells are confined to the milk ducts. *In situ* means "remaining in place." With DCIS, the cancer cells are contained within the milk ducts. Many clinicians believe we should not think of DCIS as a true cancer (as it cannot spread in its pure form), but the classification has not yet changed.
>
> Please note that lobular carcinoma *in situ* (LCIS) is not a cancer, but can raise the future risk of getting a cancer in either breast.
>
> • Invasive breast cancer
> Abnormal cells from inside the milk ducts have escaped through the duct wall into nearby breast tissue. Inflammatory breast cancer typically spreads to regional lymph nodes before diagnosis.It has the capacity to travel (through the blood stream or lymphatic vessels) from the breast to distant sites in the body, including the bone, lungs, and liver. We call this **metastasis** (meh-TAS-tah-sis).

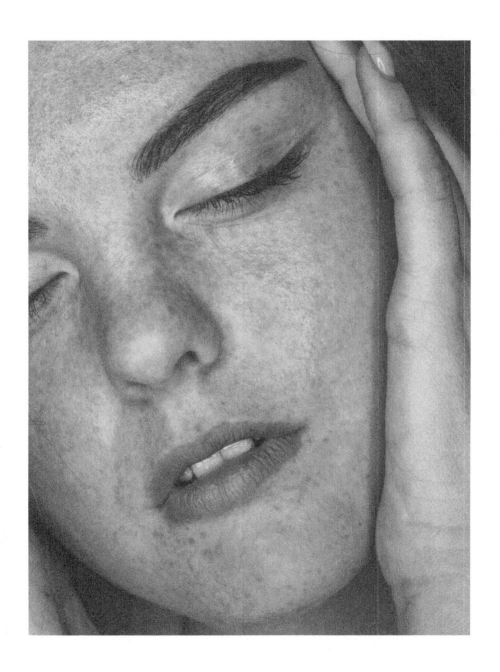

PATHOLOGY

UNDER THE MICROSCOPE

Invasive cancer

The analysis of the removed tissue can lead to several different reports. Some tests take longer than others, and not all tests may be performed by the same laboratory. Typically, you will hear some basic information in the first week after surgery, and all of the results are usually back within a few weeks. Your surgeon can let you know when the results are back, and if you don't hear from your doctor, give her a call.

There isn't just one face to breast cancer

Your doctor will order a series of tests on the cancer and nearby tissues to create a "profile" of your breast cancer. Some of these tests may be performed after the initial biopsy, while others may be done after your lumpectomy or mastectomy. Your pathology report is so important because it provides information you and your doctor need to make the appropriate personalized management choices for you.

Management decisions depend on characteristics such as:

- the size and appearance of the cancer
- how quickly the cancer is growing
- any signs of spread to nearby healthy tissues
- whether hormones (estrogen, for example) or genetic mutations (such as overexpression of HER-2) — are factors in the cancer's growth and development

What is cancer?

Cancer is a condition in which cells do not die at the normal rate. As the cell growth exceeds cell death, a mass of tissue (tumor) can form. Breast cancer happens when cells in the breast divide and grow abnormally. Many (but not all) breast cancers grow slowly and are not detected until 10 to 15 years before we can feel it. Up to 75% of breast cancers begin in the milk ducts, while 10 to 15% begin in the lobules. The remainder start in other breast tissues.

strength

61

Invasive cancer

Invasive or non-invasive?

We may conveniently divide breast cancer into two categories: Invasive versus non-invasive breast cancer. The latter is also referred to as carcinoma *in situ* (in SY-too). Only about 20 to 25% of breast cancer is non-invasive.

- **Ductal carcinoma *in situ* (DCIS)**

  A condition in which abnormal cells are confined to the milk ducts. In situ means "in place." With DCIS, the cancer cells are contained within the milk ducts. Lobular carcinoma *in situ* is not a true cancer (please see previous chapter for info on LCIS).

- **Invasive breast cancer**

  Abnormal cells from inside milk ducts have escaped through the duct wall into nearby breast tissue. While most of the time the cancer does not spread to nodes or distant organs, invasive breast cancer has the capacity to travel (through the blood stream or lymphatic vessels) from the breast to other parts of the body.

The next section typically defines the removed tissue, and if cancer is present provides information on features such as size, type, grade, hormone receptor status and whether HER2/neu is overexpressed. If the surgeon removed lymph nodes, the status of these nodes (involved with cancer, or not) should be included.

Microscopic description

Here you will find what the pathologist saw and measured when she looked at the biopsy tissue under a microscope. Tumor size is reported in centimeters (cm) or millimeters (1 inch = 2.54 cm = 25.4 mm). The optimal way to measure tumor size is under a microscope. If the length and width of the biopsy that contains cancer cells are measured, the longer of the two is reported as the tumor size.

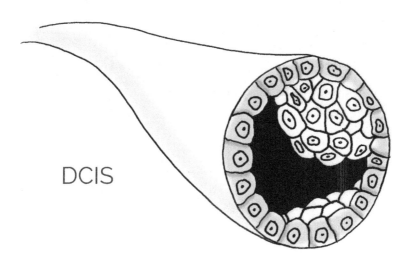

DCIS

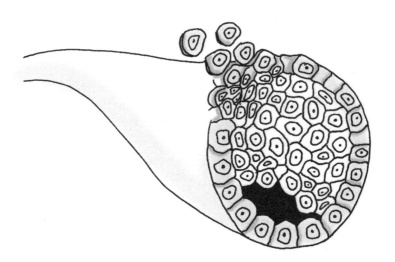

Invasive ductal

Invasive cancer

Types

Let's look at invasive breast cancer by subtype:

- Ductal   76 %
- Lobular   8 %
- Ductal/lobular   7 %
- Mucinous (colloid   2.4 %
- Tubular   1.5 %
- Medullary   1.2 %
- Papillary   1 %

Less common subtypes:

Inflammatory breast cancer
This uncommon form of breast cancer is especially aggressive. Symptoms may include swelling and redness of the breast. Sometimes the skin has an orange peel-like appearance (peau d'orange).

Paget disease of the breast (uncommon)
Here, the abnormal cells are in the skin in or around the nipple. There may be an associated underlying mass in the breast.

Metaplastic breast cancer
This a rare cancer can be hard to diagnose. These tumors tend to be larger and have a higher tumor grade.

Angiosarcoma
This rare cancer begins in cells that line blood or lymph vessels. This cancer sometimes develops 5 to 10 years (or more) later as a complication of previous radiation treatment. Angiosarcoma can also occur in individuals who develop lymphedema as a result of lymph node surgery and/or radiation therapy to manage breast cancer. Unfortunately, angiosarcomas tend to grow and can spread quickly.

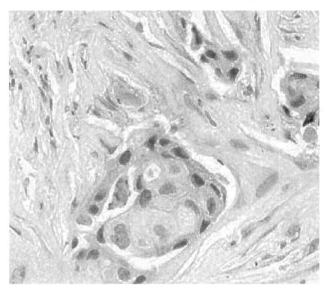

Ductal
(cords and nests of tumor cells)

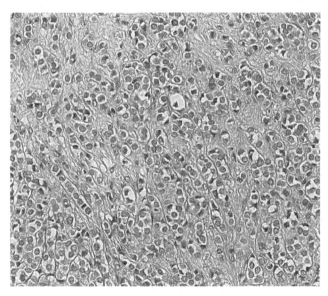

Lobular
Small cancer cells grow in a single file. LCIS is present in two-thirds of cases (DCIS may also join)

Invasive cancer

Grade

Tumor grade* is a description of a cancer (as seen under a microscope), based on how abnormal/aggressive the cells appear. Using a microscope, the pathologist examines the tissue removed from your body. She then decides if the cells are benign (not cancer) or malignant (cancer). Grade 1 (low-grade) is the least aggressive, and grade 3 (high-grade) the most.

Nottingham grade

This system grades tumors based on tubule/duct formation, nuclear grade, and mitotic (cell division) rate. Each of these factors is assigned a score from 1 to 3 (1 is best). We then add the scores to get a total of 3 to 9, with 9 being the most aggressive. In general, a lower grade means a better prognosis. As inflammatory breast cancer is aggressive, management for non-metastatic disease includes drugs such as chemotherapy, breast removal, underarm node dissection, and radiation therapy.

- Tubule formation
How close to normal do the breast (milk) duct structures appear?

- Nuclear grade
An evaluation of the size and shape of the cancer cell nucleus

- Mitotic rate (how fast is cancer growing?)
How many dividing cells are present in the microscope field?

Putting it all together

Total score 3 to 5: Low-grade (relatively non-aggressive); well-differentiated
Total score 6 or 7: Intermediate-grade; moderately differentiated
Total score 8 or 9: High-grade (aggressive); poorly-differentiated

---

* Cancer grade is *not* the same as cancer stage. Cancer stage refers to the size and extent of the cancer, and whether the cancer has spread.

Rate of cell growth

Your pathology report may have information about the rate of cell growth — what proportion of the cancer cells within the tumor are growing and dividing to form new cancer cells. A higher percentage points to a faster-growing, more aggressive cancer. Here are two tests that are sometimes used to determine the cell growth rate:

- **Ki-67**

This cell protein increases as cells prepare to divide and multiply. A staining process can measure the percentage of tumor cells that are positive for Ki-67. The more positive cells there are, the the faster the growth rate. In breast cancer, a result of less than 10% is considered low, 10-20% intermediate, and high if greater than 20%.

- **S-phase**

This number tells you what percentage of cells in the sample are in the process of copying their genetic information (DNA). S-phase, short for "synthesis phase," happens right before a cell divides into two new cells. A result of less than 6% is considered low, 6-10% intermediate, and more than 10% is considered high.

Experts don't agree on how to use the results of these tests when making management decisions. As a result, not all doctors order these tests routinely, so don't be alarmed if they are not in your pathology report.

Lymphvascular invasion (LVI)

Lymphvascular (angiolymphatic) invasion, or LVI means that there are cancer cells in the small lymph or blood vessels that drain lymph fluid and blood from your breast, ultimately into your circulation system. Please note that lymphatic or vascular (blood) invasion is different from lymph node involvement.

A hallmark of inflammatory breast cancer is the presence of small bits of tumor in the small lymphatic channels of the breast skin.

Margins

noun mar·gin \ˈmär-jin\
a rim of normal breast tissue surrounding a suspicious area

A mastectomy (breast removal) with a dissection of axillary (underarm) lymph nodes is a vital part of the management of inflammatory breast cancer. It is typically performed after the completion of chemotherapy-containing systemic therapy. The goal of surgery is to remove all known cancer. Given the high chance the cancer can come back in the local area, a skin-sparing mastectomy is generally *not* offered.

At mastectomy, we hope to not have the cancer extending all the way to the edge of the removed specimen. If it does, we call this an involved or positive margin.

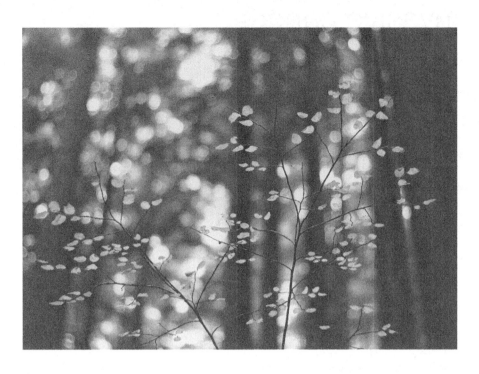

Invasive cancer

Nodes

If your surgeon removes lymph nodes (for example, axillary ones in the underarm area), the pathologist examines the removed material to determine whether or not they contain cancer.

- **Lymph node-negative:** Nodes don't contain cancer.

- **Lymph node-positive:** Nodes contain cancer.

Cancer that is confined to the breast (and *not* spreading to regional nodes) has the best prognosis, in general. The more lymph nodes that contain cancer, the poorer the prognosis tends to be.

Inflammatory breast cancer

For inflammatory breast cancer, an aggressive form of locally advanced breast cancer (LABC), **nearly all patients will have lymph node involvement at the time of diagnosis,** and appropixately 36 percent will have identifiable distant spread (metastasis) of cancer.

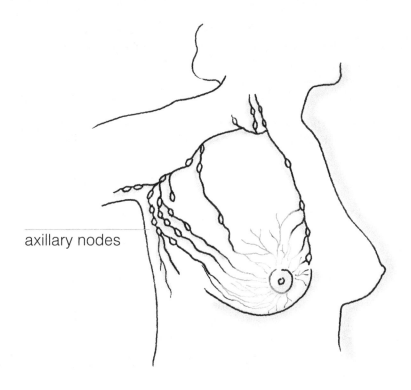

axillary nodes

Axillary Lymph Nodes

Four or more nodes involved (prior to treatment) is associated with poorer outcomes among those with inflammatory breast cancer.

Invasive cancer

Estrogen receptors (ER)

Your biopsy or surgical material will be tested to see if your breast cancer cells have receptors for the hormones estrogen and progesterone. Hormone receptors are proteins — found in and on breast cells — that pick up hormone signals telling the cells to grow.

A cancer is estrogen receptor-positive (or ER+) if it has receptors for estrogen. This suggests that cancer cells, like normal breast cells, receive signals from estrogen that promote growth. The cancer is progesterone receptor-positive (PR+) if it has progesterone receptors; that is, the cancer cells receive signals from progesterone that promote their growth. **For those with inflammatory breast cancer, 44 percent are estrogen receptor positive, and 30 percent are progesterone receptor positive.**

Why is ER/PR status important?

Hormone receptor status indicates whether your cancer is likely to respond to endocrine (anti-hormonal) therapy. Endocrine therapy approaches include medications that either (1) lower the amount of estrogen in your body or (2) block estrogen from supporting the growth and function of breast cells. If the breast cancer cells have hormone receptors, these medications can slow or stop their growth. If the cancer is hormone-receptor-negative (no receptors are present), then hormonal therapy would not work. You and your doctor can then select other types of treatment.

ER/PR: Understanding your results

A test should be done for both estrogen and progesterone receptors (ER/PR). If your result is reported as "positive" or "negative," ask your doctor for a specific number. Breast cancers that have at least 1 percent of cells staining positive for ER should be considered ER-positive. Even cancers with low numbers of hormone receptors may respond to hormonal therapy.

ESTROGEN hormone fuels the growth and division of some breast cancer cells

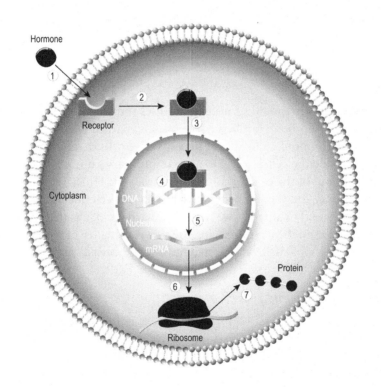

Invasive cancer

ER/PR

Estrogen and progesterone receptors are scored from 0 (no receptors) to 100 (all of your cancer cells appear to have receptors). A score of "0" generally means that hormonal therapy will not be helpful in treating the breast cancer. When the score is 0, the cancer is called hormone-receptor-negative. The alternative Allred system scores the ER from 0 to 8, the higher the better. Sometimes, a report will come back from the laboratory saying that the hormone status is "unknown." If you receive a result of "unknown," ask your doctor what this means, and ask what further steps should be taken to determine your hormone receptor status.

HER-2

Invasive breast cancers should be tested for HER2 (human epidermal growth factor receptor-2), a protein on the surface of cells charged with stimulating cell growth and repair. About 15 to 20% of patients have cells that have an excess of HER-2 genes inside the cell, leading to an extraordinary number of HER-2 receptors sticking out of the cell like antennae. These exra HER2 receptors receive a growth hormone, and then transmit a signal into the cell nucleus to make the cell more aggressive. Fortunately, we recently developed drugs that target the HER-2 pathway, dramatically improving the survival chance of patients with HER-2 overexpression. HER2 is reported for invasive breast cancer (not typically for DCIS or LCIS). Here are two common tests for HER2:

- *Immunohistochemistry (IHC)*

Detects the amount of HER2 protein on the surface of the cancer cells. IHC is often the first test done. If the IHC score is 0 or 1+, there is no HER-2 overexpression (HER-2 negative); if the score is 3+, there is overexpression (HER-2 positive); if the IHC score is 2+, the test is equivocal, and we move to FISH testing.

- *Fluorescence in situ hybridization (FISH) testing*

Detects the number of HER2/neu genes in the cancer cell. FISH is typically scored as positive or negative for HER2 overexpression. If the answer is not clear, an IHC test may be done (please see above).

74

Estrogen & Progesterone Receptors

(Inflammatory breast cancer)

ER +	44%	Cancer cells have hormone receptors for estrogen and progesterone. These hormones support cancer growth.
PR +	30%	Progesterone (a so-called female hormone) is helping to support growth of the cancer cell.

Invasive cancer

HER2

Breast cancer is best thought of not as a single entity, but rather as a variety of diseases. Even breast cancers that appear similar under the microscope may have very different "personalities," or genetic fingerprints. HER2 overexpressing (HER2 positive) breast cancer is one subtype. Unfortunately, when cells are HER2 positive, they tend to be more aggressive.

HER2 function

All of our cells have a life cycle, one that is typically lived in an orderly fashion. This normalcy can be disrupted by either events within (or from outside) the cell. We all have HER2 genes designed to make HER2 protein. When two copies of the gene are present in normal amounts, the protein helps with cell growth and development. The HER2 protein transmits signals from outside the cell to the nucleus inside the cell. Growth factors — chemicals that carry growth-regulating orders — attach to the HER2 protein and signal normal cell growth.

HER2 positive

HER2 is a normal gene; however, when amplified (there are too many), it causes cancer and is called an oncogene. Many scientists had postulated that oncogenes were related to growth factors. In the early 1980s, a Genentech scientist, a British protein chemist, and an Israeli protein expert together proved that growth factors are related to cancer. They found an oncogene that was a mutated form of the epidermal growth factor (EGF) cell-surface receptor gene. By linking the study of cell-growth signals and cancer, this finding explained how an oncogene worked.

A healthy cell contains a normal quantity of approximately 20,000 of HER2 proteins (or receptors) on the cell surface. Because of HER2 gene amplification, HER2-positive cancer cells have an abundance of HER2 receptors on the cell surface (approximately 2 million, or 100 times more than a healthy cell), leading to uncontrolled cancer cell growth. Up to 1 in 4 individuals with breast cancer are HER2-positive, a more aggressive form of the disease.

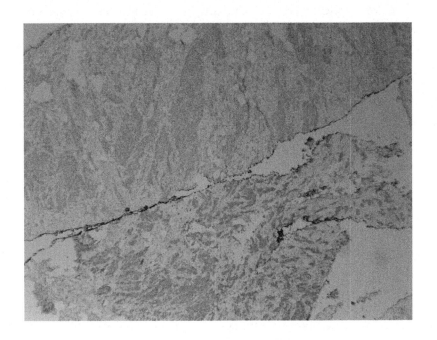

HER2

Some cancers are heterogeneous. The top part of the illustration shows no overexpression of HER-2, while the bottom part has overexpression (cells stain dark brown)

Invasive

HER2

Dysregulation of ERBB2 (HER2) signaling in cancer involves an excess of signals that stimulate cancer cells to grow and spread.

1 *Amplify (genes)*

Up to 20 to 25% of individuals with breast cancer have cancer cells with too many copies of the HER2 gene. This results in an overabundance of HER-2 receptors (which stick out like antennae) on the cell surface.

2 *Dimerize*

The HER family sits on the cell surface. We have HER1 (EGFR), HER2 (ERBB2), HER3, and HER4. While each of them can bind (dimerize) to one of the others, HER2 is the preferred bonding partner. HER2 does not need an outside stimulant; it aids in activating a signal by binding with one of the other type of HER receptors. HER2 exists in an open conformation that makes it always ready to dimerize. HER2-containing dimers have increased signaling potency relative to dimers that do not contain HER2, as HER2 is able to decrease the rate of disconnection from its dimerized partner.

3 *Send the signal*

As described above, HER family receptors are activated by ligand-induced dimerization, or receptor pairing. It is as if the HER family members grap arms with another member if the first is stimulated by a growth hormone. Once the pair (now known as a HER dimer) is created, the downstream signalling process begins. Signalling pathways include the so-called MAPK proliferation and the PI3K/Akt pro-survival pathways.

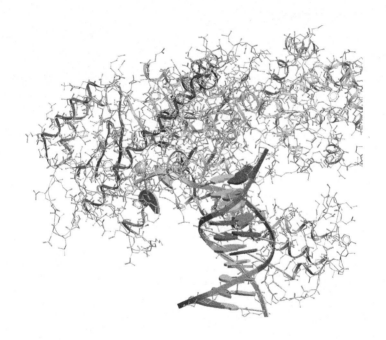

Inappropriate signaling from HER2 can lead to:

- Increased/uncontrolled cell growth
- Decreased apoptosis (programmed cell suicide)
- Enhanced cancer cell movement
- Angiogenesis (formation of new blood vessels)

Invasive cancer

Molecular fingerprint

Breast cancer is a group of diseases that may be conveniently divided into at least three subtypes, based on the presence or absence of molecular markers for estrogen or progesterone receptors and human epidermal growth factor 2 (ERBB2):

- Hormone receptor (estrogen receptor and/or progesterone receptor positive) *and* HER2 (ERBB2) negative
- HER2 (ERBB2) positive
- Triple negative (estrogen- and/or progesterone-receptor negative)

There is an alternative classification system, in which breast cancer is divided into at least four distinct molecular subtypes:

- Luminal A-like (best prognosis)
- Luminal B-like
- HER2-like
- Basal like (triple negative/basal-like) (worst prognosis))

These same subtypes also appear in ductal carcinoma *in situ*. Breast cancers that do not fall into any of these subtypes are often listed as unclassified.

Okay, I know my cancer's ER, PR, HER2, and grade. Now what?

Systemic treatment decisions and prognosis are heavily influenced by stage, and cancer characteristics such as estrogen receptor status (ER), HER2 status, and grade.

	ER or PR positive *and* ERBB2 -	ERBB2+ (HER2 +)	Triple-negative
What	1% or more of cells positive for estrogen receptors (ER) or progesterone receptors (PR)	Cancer stains strongly for ERBB2 (3+) or ERBB2 gene is amplified.	Tumor *not* positive for estrogen receptor, progesterone receptor, or ERBB2
How	Estrogen receptor activates cancer growth pathways	Oncogene ERBB2 overactive	Unknown (likely various ways)

Ask

- **Where**

  Where is my cancer located in the breast? Has it spread to regional nodes or to distant sites (metastasized)?

- **What**

  Can you explain my pathology report to me? Is my breast cancer hormone receptor positive or HER2 positive? What does that mean for me?

- **Copies**

  Can I have a copy of my pathology report?

- **Second opinions**

  Most insurance plans will allow you to get an additional opinion, as long as the second health care provider is a member of your health plan. Sometimes that opinion is best obtained from an expert in pathology, reviewing the slides containing the material from your surgery. Still, inflammatory breast cancer diagnosis is largely based on what we see on physical exam, and we need to move with all due deliberate speed into treatment.

  You should ask if there are any **clinical trials** for inflammatory breast cancer that are appropriate for you.

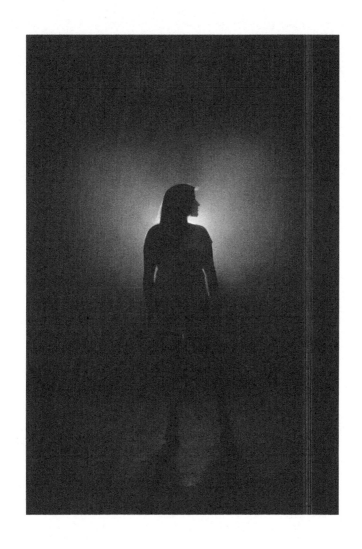

STAGE

CANCER EXTENT

Stage

The stage describes the **extent of cancer** in the body. For inflammatory breast cancer, if there is spread to distant organs, we label it Stage IV; if the cancer is confined to the breast and regional lymph nodes, it is either Stage IIIB or IIIC. Stage is one of the most important factors in determining prognosis and management options. Staging provides a common language for health care team members to effectively communicate about a patient's cancer and to collaborate on the best courses of management. Understanding the cancer's stage is also critical to identifying clinical trials that may be appropriate for particular patients.

Testing

Depending on the results of your physical exam and biopsy, your doctor may want you to have certain imaging tests such as a chest x-ray, mammograms of both breasts, bone scans, computed tomography (CT) scans, magnetic resonance imaging (MRI), and/or positron emission tomography (PET) scans. Blood tests may also be done to evaluate your overall health and can uncommonly indicate if the cancer has spread to certain organs.

TNM (T is for Tumor, N is for Nodes, M is for Metastases)

We use a staging system that allows us to summarize the extent of cancer in a clear way. The most common system used to describe the stages of breast cancer is the American Joint Committee on Cancer (AJCC) TNM system.

- **Clinical Stage**

Your clinical stage is based on your physical exam, biopsy, and imaging.

- **Pathologic stage**

Your pathologic stage uses information from the clinical stage, but adds in the findings from surgery (for example, how many lymph nodes are involved with cancer, if any nodes were removed).

Staging

Metastases (distant spread of cancer)

Symptoms can include significant weight loss, unusual bone pain, a chronic cough, and shortness of breath can be symptoms of metastases.

Testing

- Bone scan or sodium fluoride PET/CT scan
- CT scan (chest, abdomen, and pelvis)
- FDG Positron Emission Tomography (PET) scan (optional)
- Genetic counseling, if you are at risk for hereditary breast cancer

The stages of breast cancer range from 0 to IV (0 to 4). We determine the overall stage by looking at three factors:

- **T** (Tumor size)
- **N** (Lymph node status)
- **M** (Metastases)

For example, an individual with a T1 tumor (less than 2 cm, or under 4/5"), no lymph nodes with cancer (N0) and no metastases (M0) is Stage IA (T1, N0, M0). The higher the stage, the poorer the prognosis. The highest stage (Stage IV) is any cancer that has metastases (M1).

- Clinical staging is determined before surgery
- Pathologic staging is determined after surgery

T is for Tumor (T4d)

TX: Stage cannot be assessed	
T0: No tumor found	
Tis: Carcinoma *in situ* (*in situ* means remaining in place)	**Tis (DCIS):** Ductal carcinoma *in situ* **Tis (Paget):** Paget disease of the nipple
T1: Tumor 2 cm or less	**T1mi:** 0.1 cm or smaller **T1a:** Larger than 0.1 cm, but no larger than 0.5 cm **T1b:** Larger than 0.5 cm, but no larger than 1 cm **T1c:** Larger than 1 cm, but no larger than 2 cm
T2: Tumor over 2 cm, but no larger than 5 cm	
T3: Tumor over 5 cm	
T4: Tumor any size, but has spread beyond the breast to the chest wall and/or skin	**T4a:** Tumor spread to the chest wall **T4b:** Tumor spread to the skin, but is not inflammatory breast cancer **T4c:** Tumor spread to the chest wall *and* skin **T4d: Inflammatory breast cancer**

N is for Nodes
Clinical (before surgery)

NX: Regional nodes cannot be assessed (e.g., they were previously removed)

N0: No regional node metastases

N1: Metastases to movable ipsilateral level I, II axillary node(s)

N2a: Spread to ipsilateral level I, II axillary nodes fixed to one another (matted) or to other structures

N2b: Spread to ipsilateral internal mammary nodes
and in the absence of clinically evident level I, II axillary node metastases

N3a Spread to ipsilateral infraclavicular lymph node(s)

N3b Spread to ipsilateral internal mammary lymph node(s) and axillary node(s)

N3c Metastases in ipsilateral supraclavicular (above collar bone) node(s)

N is for Nodes
Pathologic (after surgery)

pNX Regional nodes cannot be assessed

pN0 Cancer has not spread to nearby nodes*

pN1mi: Micrometastases (tiny areas of cancer spread) in 1 to 3 lymph nodes under the arm. The areas of cancer spread in the lymph nodes are 2 mm or less across (but at least 200 cancer cells or 0.2mm across).

pN1a: Cancer spread to 1 to 3 nodes under the arm with at least one area of cancer spread greater than 2 mm across.

pN1b: Cancer spread to internal mammary nodes, but spread only in sentinel node biopsy (it did not cause the nodes to become enlarged).

pN1c: Both N1a and N1b apply.

pN2a: Cancer spread to 4 to 9 lymph nodes under the arm, with at least one area of cancer spread larger than 2 mm.

pN2b: Cancer spread to one or more internal mammary lymph nodes, causing them to become enlarged.

pN3a: Cancer spread to 10 or more axillary lymph nodes, with at least one area of cancer spread greater than 2mm, or cancer has spread to the lymph nodes under the collarbone, with at least one area of cancer spread over 2mm.

pN3b: Cancer in at least one axillary node (with at least one area of cancer spread greater than 2 mm) and in internal mammary lymph nodes, or cancer spread to 4 or more axillary lymph nodes (with at least one area of cancer spread greater than 2 mm), and tiny amounts of cancer are found in internal mammary nodes on sentinel lymph node biopsy.

pN3c: Cancer has spread to the nodes above the collarbone with at least one area of cancer spread greater than 2mm.

M is for Metastasis

M0: No distant spread is found on x-rays (or other imaging procedures) or by physical exam.*

M1: Cancer has spread to distant organs. The most common sites are bone, lung, and liver, and brain.

* before surgery

Staging following neoadjuvant* therapy is designated with **"yc" or "yp"** prefix to the T and N classification. There is no anatomic stage group assigned if there is a complete pathological response (pCR) to neoadjuvant therapy; for example, ypT0, ypN0, cM0.

Inflammatory = Stage III

Locally advanced breast cancer			
Stage IIIA	T0	N2	M0
	T1	N2	M0
	T2	N2	M0
	T3	N1	M0
	T3	N2	M0
Stage IIIB	**T4**	**N0**	**M0**
	T4	**N1**	**M0**
	T4	**N2**	**M0**
Stage IIIC	**Any T**	**N3**	**M0**
Metastatic breast cancer			
Stage IV	Any T	Any N	M1

Inflammatory breast cancer that has not spread to distant sites (such as the bone, liver, or lungs) is generally considered to be Stage IIIB upon initial diagnosis. If it has spread outside the breast and lymph node regions, it may be diagnosed as Stage IV.

Stage IIIB

The inflammatory breast cancer may or may not have spread to the axillary (underarm) or internal mammary nodes (next to the breast bone). It has not spread to distant sites of the body (T4, N0-2, M0).

Stage IIIC

The inflammatory breast cancer has spread to 10 or more axillary lymph nodes, the internal mammary nodes, and/or nodes around the collarbone. It has not spread to distant sites of the body.

Metastases

For locally advanced breast cancer (including the inflammatory type), tests are done to check for cancer spread to distant organs such as the bones, lungs or liver). Although the cancer starts in the breast, it can travel to other parts of the body through the lymph fluid and/or the blood. If your breast cancer has spread, the prognosis is poorer.

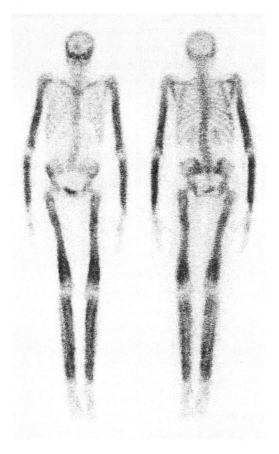

Metastasis
Cancer spread to distant organs, such as the bones, lungs or liver.

Staging

New and improved system

In 2017, the American Joint Committee on Cancer (AJCC) updated the staging system for breast cancer. **Stage** refers to the amount of cancer (size of the main tumor, spread to lymph nodes or to distant sites). Now, the definitions of each stage vary depending on cancer type. Cancer stage often correlates with outcomes, and management recommendations usually take into account the stage of disease.

Incorporating cancer cell biology

As our knowledge of tumor biology increases, it has become clear that stage is not the only factor that impacts prognosis. Tumor biology and behavior are very important, and in some cases may be more important than stage. A small tumor with aggressive behavior characteristics may may result in worse outcomes compared to a larger, but slower growing cancer.

Prognostic stage group

The 8th version of the AJCC staging system for breast cancer now takes into account tumor biology. Factors such as cell grade, estrogen receptor and HER2 status, grade, and (if performed) tumor genomic tests such as OncoType DX are now incorporated into the clinical (before surgery) and pathological (after surgery) prognostic stage. Taking into account these biologic factors means that the stage will have more meaningful prognostic information. In a large validation study performed by researchers at the University of Texas MD Anderson Cancer Center, 31% of patients were upstaged, and 20% of patients were downstaged. The updated prognostic stage performed better (in terms of predicting patient outcomes) than the standard anatomic stage.

The pathologic prognostic stage is not applicable to patients receiving neoadjuvant therapy. **Patients with localized inflammatory breast cancer typically receive neoadjuvant chemotherapy, and the new Prognostic Stage Grouping does not apply.**

Anatomic Prognostic Stage Group

TNM	Grade	HER2	ER	PR	Prognostic Group
	G1	Positive	Positive	Positive	**IIIA**
				Negative	**IIIB**
			Negative	Any	**IIIB**
		Negative	Positive	Positive	**IIIA**
				Negative	**IIIB**
			Negative	Any	**IIIB**
	G2	Positive	Positive	Positive	**IIIA**
T4 N0 M0				Negative	**IIIB**
T4 N1 ** **M0**			Negative	Any	**IIIB**
T4 N2 M0		Negative	Positive	Positive	**IIIA**
Any T N3 M0				Negative	**IIIB**
			Negative	Negative	**IIIC**
			Negaitve	Positive	**IIIB**
	G3	Positive	Any	Any	**IIIB**
		Negative	Positive	Positive	
				Negative	**IIIC**
			Negative	Any	
Any T Any N M1	Any	Any	Any	Any	**IV**

* N1 does not include N1mi. T1, N1mi, M0 and T0, N1mi, M0 are included for prognostic staging with T1, N0, M0 cancers of the same prognostic factor status.

** N1 includes N1mi. T2, T3, and T4 cancers and N1mi are included for prognostic staging with T2, N1; T3, N1; and T4, N1, respectively.

Note: If performed, when OncoType DX score is less than 11 for T1-2, N0, M0 disease, if HER 2 negative, the Pathologic Prognostic Group is IA.

PROGNOSIS

Inflammatory

Prognosis

With appropriately aggressive treatment, up to 62 percent of those with IBC will live at least five years and 41 to 47 percent will have no signs of breast cancer 10 years after diagnosis. While these rates are not nearly as high as for other types of breast cancer, new treatments continue to improve survival.

Inflammatory, non-metastatic: Median survival 57 months

Let's look at survival in a different way: Median survival is the length of time for half of the patients in a group to have died. By definition, half of the patients in that group are still alive. The US Surveillance, Epidemiology, and End Results (SEER) database shows that for Stage III inflammatory breast cancer, the **median survival is on the order of 57 months.** These numbers are a bit outdated, however. Recent advancements in research and treatment are leading to better survival rates for women with inflammatory breast cancer. Each person's cancer and treatment are unique to them and these statistics do not reflect how you as an individual person will respond to treatment.

Survival rates improving

With modern treatment, the survival rate is much higher than in the past. An analysis from the Surveillance, Epidemiology, and End Results (SEER) database demonstrated 20-year cancer-specific survival of 20 versus 9 percent for patients with IBC treated in 1995 compared with 1975. Despite these improvements, the survival rate for patients with IBC remains significantly worse compared with women with non-inflammatory, locally advanced breast cancer. For Stage IV, the median survival drops to 21 months.

Poor prognostic features

Poor prognostic features include triple-negative receptor status, hormone receptor-positive/human epidermal growth factor receptor 2 (HER2)-negative status, four or more involved nodes prior to treatment, and lack of response to neoadjuvant (before surgery) chemotherapy.

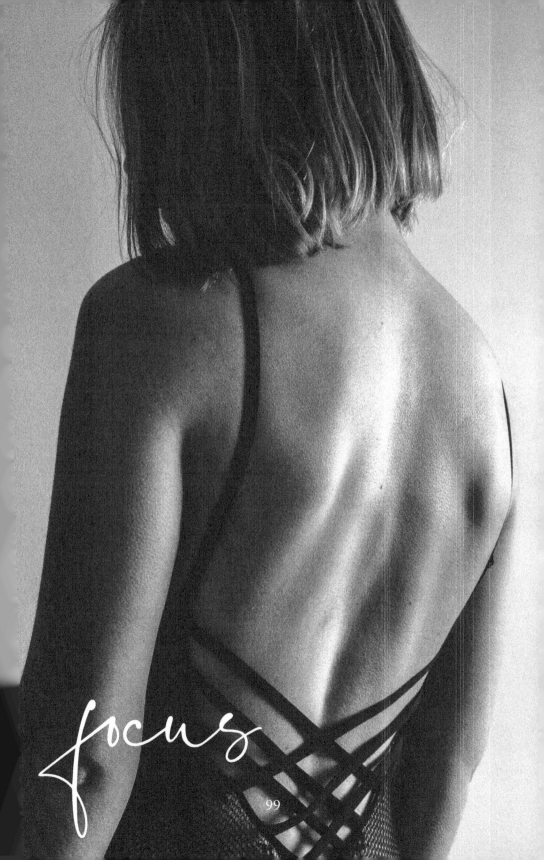

focus

MANAGEMENT
OVERVIEW

Invasive

Management: An Overview

In this chapter, I hope to explain the types of treatment tools that represent the best treatment for inflammatory breast cancer. As you make treatment decisions, I encourage you to consider clinical trials as an option. **Clinical trials** are research studies that test a new approach to management.

I designed this chapter to give you a brief overview of the intense management recommended for inflammatory breast cancer. Over the next several chapters, we will explore the various treatment modalities (chemotherapy, surgery, radiation therapy, and more) in more detail.

Multiple treatment types

For the management of inflammatory breast cancer, doctors specializing in varying areas of cancer management work together to create your overall treatment plan. This multidisciplinary team includes a variety of physicians, as well as other health care professionals, and may include physician assistants, oncology nurses, pharmacists, dieticians, counselors, and others.

Localized inflammatory breast cancer is typically managed with a combination of strategies, including chemotherapy, surgery, radiation therapy, and (sometimes) targeted therapies. This combined modality approach has led to better control of inflammatory breast cancer than had been possible in the past. One hallmark of IBC management is the use of chemotherapy *before* surgery.

Distant spread (metastasis)

Approximately 5% of patients will have simultaneous metastatic disease identified at initial presentation. For more details on the meaning of T, N, and M, please go to chapter 5 (breast cancer staging). Care for those with distant spread of cancer is individualized, with drugs such as chemotherapy often the main approach. Surgery and radiation therapy may be selectively offered.

Invasive

Management: Initial evaluation

The diagnosis of breast cancer is based on clinical examination in combination with imaging, and confirmed by pathological assessment such as a biopsy (tissue sampling).

Guidelines

The National Comprehensive Cancer Network (www.nccn.org) offers recommendations for the initial workup of patients with early breast cancer. Here are the January 2019 recommendations:

- History and physical exam
- Blood tests (complete blood cell; comprehensive metabolic panel, including liver function tests and alkaline phosphatase).
- Diagnostic bilateral mammograms
- Pathology review
- Determination of tumor estrogen receptor (ER) status. The progesterone receptor (PR), and HER2 status should also be checked.
- Genetic counseling if you are at high-risk for hereditary breast cancer
- Fertility counseling (if pre-menopausal)
- Bone scan or sodium fluoride PET/CT scan
- CT scan with contrast (chest/abdomen/pelvis)
- FDG PET/CT (optional)
- Breast MRI (optional)

Cancer spread (metastasis)

Approximately 30 percent of patients with inflammatory breast cancer will present with cancer spread (metastasis) to distant sites such as the bones, liver, lungs, or brain. If metastases are present, the disease is Stage IV breast cancer. We will review the management of **metastatic breast cancer** in Chapter 12.

Invasive

Management: Genetic counseling

I want to make a brief detour to talk a bit about genetic counseling, We will go in more detail in a later chapter. Might you be a candidate for genetic testing?

You have breast cancer and ...	• you have have a known mutation (in the family) of a gene that increases cancer risk • you are 50 or under • you are 60 or under with ER/PR/HER2 negative breast cancer • you have 2 breast cancers* • you are of Ashkenazi Jewish descent • you are male • you have 1+ close blood relatives with breast cancer found at 50 years or younger (or with ovarian, fallopian, or primary peritoneal cancer); 2 or more close blood relatives with breast, pancreas and/or prostate cancer (Gleason score 7 or higher)
You have a personal history of **ovarian cancer**	

Other criteria include a personal and/or family history of at least three of the following:

- Breast, pancreas, prostate (Gleason score 7+), diffuse stomach (gastric), colon, endometrial, thyroid, or kidney cancer, melanoma, sarcoma, adrenocortical carcinoma, brain tumors, or leukemia

- Skin problems consistent with Cowden syndrome

- Macrocephaly, hamartomatous polyps of the gastrointestinal tract

---

* bilateral disease or at least two separate cancers in the same breast

BRCA

Breast cancer genes (basics)

Patients at high risk for having hereditary (inherited) breast cancer should receive **genetics counseling.** Approximately 5% to 10% of breast cancer patients have an inherited genetic mutation. The most common mutations (mistakes) associated with breast cancer are ones in tumor suppression genes BRCA1 and BRCA2 (BReast CAncer genes #1 and #2). You may recall that the actress Angelina Jolie had a BRCA mutation.

Breast cancer risk
Approximately 12 percent of women in the general population will develop breast cancer during their lives. By contrast, 72 percent of women who inherit a harmful BRCA1 mutation and around 69 percent of women who inherit a harmful BRCA2 mutation will develop breast cancer by 80 years of age. In addition, breast cancer incidence rises in early adulthood until 30 to 40 years for BRCA1 carriers, and until 40 to 50 years for BRCA2 carriers, after which it plateaus at 20 to 30 per 1000 person years until at least age 80. BRCA1 carriers are more likely to develop a so-called triple negative breast cancer, an especially aggressive form of the disease.

Ovarian cancer risk
About 1.3 percent of women in the general population will develop ovarian cancer sometime during their lives. By contrast, 44 percent of women who inherit a harmful BRCA1 mutation (and 17 percent of women who inherit a harmful BRCA2 mutation) will develop ovarian cancer by age 70 years.

BRCA mutations increase risk of other cancers, too
The incidence may increase for cancer of the opposite breast, colon (BRCA1; amount uncertain), male prostate cancer (BRCA2 may increase risk 5- to 9-fold; the magnitude of increase for BRCA1 carriers is not well-understood), and pancreas cancer (BRCA1 unclear; BRCA2 5 percent, compared to 1.5 percent in the general population). We are learning about the risk of stomach and biliary cancer (BRCA2), skin or uveal (eye) melanoma for those with BRCA2 mutations, fallopian tube cancer (lifetime risk about 0.6 percent), uterine papillary serious carcinoma, and others.

Treatment

Systemic therapy (including chemotherapy) first

For most breast cancer types, treatment often begins with surgery. However, for inflammatory breast cancer (IBC), treatment usually starts with chemotherapy. The treatment of IBC should involve a **combined modality approach,** including systemic therapy (such as chemotherapy), followed by surgery (breast removal/mastectomy) and radiation therapy. Selected patients may then take pills designed to reduce exposure of the cancer to estrogen.

Preoperative (neoadjuvant) chemotherapy

Unfortunately, we do not have high level evidence (such as large randomized clinical trials) telling us which chemotherapy drugs are optimal for the management of inflammatory breast cancer, since the disease is so uncommon. In that context, your medical oncologist will turn to the available data.

Why follow chemotherapy with surgery?

A retrospective analysis of the benefits of preoperative chemotherapy followed by mastectomy over chemotherapy alone showed **lower local recurrence rates and longer breast cancer-specific survival.** Here are the results from a large retrospective study of patients with inflammatory breast cancer managed at the University of Texas (USA) M.D. Anderson Cancer Center: Using chemotherapy (in this case doxorubicin/Adriamycin-based, followed by radiation therapy, mastectomy, or both) and additional chemotherapy following surgery led to a 15-year disease-free survival of 28 percent.

Is more intense chemotherapy better?

A retrospective study from Dr. Cristofanelli and colleagues at M.D. Anderson illustrates the value of adding a taxane (such as paclitaxel, or Taxol) to an anthracycline drug such as doxorubicin/Adriamycin, at least for those with estrogen-receptor negative inflammatory breast cancer. In addition, a systematic review demonstrated **better outcomes associated with more intensive systemic therapy before surgery,** at least in terms of a pathologic complete response (pCR: no residual cancer found at surgery).

team

Treatment

Systemic therapy

Chemotherapy involves the use of drugs to control or kill cells within the breast and any that may have spread to regional lymph nodes, or other parts of the body. Such disease can be microscopic, and undetectable using routine tests. Chemotherapy is usually given in cycles, over a 3 to 6 month period.

Does a complete response matter? Yes.

For those who achieve a disappearance of their cancer in the underarm/axillary lymph nodes, the overall and disease-free survival odds are better, as compared to those who have residual cancer in the axillary nodes.

If you are among the nearly 50 percent of patients (treated with an aggressive chemotherapy regimen) who have all of the cancer in the nodes go away, the prognosis is very good; **the 5 year overall survival odds for those with no residual disease in nodes are 82.5 percent,** and the relapse-free survival odds are 79 percent. In contrast, for those who have residual cancer in the regional lymph nodes, the 5 year survival odds are 37 percent, and the relapse-free survival chances 25 percent, respectively.

Guideline-based management

The National Comprehensive Cancer Network (www.nccn.org) recommends systemic therapy before surgery. The drugs should include a so-called anthracycline (for example, doxorubicin/Adriamycin), with or without taxane chemotherapy for the initial treatment of patients with inflammatory breast cancer. The NCCN panel also recommends completing the planned chemotherapy prior to breast removal (mastectomy). If the chemotherapy was not completed before surgery, it should be completed after it.

Targeted therapy

Is you cancer hormone-receptor positive? What I mean to ask is whether the cancer feeds on estrogen and/or progesterone (estrogen- and/or progesterone receptor positive). If yes, you should receive so-called endocrine therapy (tamoxifen is one example; aromatase inhibitors such as anastrazole is another) after completion of chemotherapy.

About one quarter (perhaps a bit higher for IBC) of cancers have too many HER2 receptors sticking out like antennae from the cancer cell surface. We call this HER2-positive or HER2-overexpressing, and it is associated with a poorer prognosis. However, the use of drugs targeting the HER2 pathway has substantially improved outcomes; for example the addition of traztazumab (Herceptin) to chemotherapy significantly improves response rates. Herceptin is typically given for a total of up to one year. It may be given at the same time as radiation therapy or endocrine therapy, if indicated.

For example, a research study randomized women with locally advanced breast cancer, some with the inflammatory type, to receive chemotherapy (with or without trastazumab for a year) before surgery. **The addition of trastazumab significantly improved event-free survival for patients with HER2-positive breast cancers,** with the 3-year event-free survival 71 percent, compared to 56 percent for the no trastazumab group. The researchers noted that the trastazumab was well-tolerated and, despite it being given concurrently with the chemotherapy doxorubicin/Adriamycin, led to only 2 percent of patients developing symptomatic heart failure (both of these patients responded to heart drugs).

Other HER2-targeting drugs

We have emerging evidence to suggest that other HER2-targeting drugs such as lapatinib and pertuzumab may benefit those with inflammatory breast cancer. As an example, the NEOSPHERE trial that included patients with inflammatory breast cancer demonstrated a higher pathologic complete response (no residual cancer found at surgery). Thus selected patients may have pertuzumab incorporated in the preoperative setting for HER2-positive inflammatory breast cancer.

After chemotherapy, before surgery

You should have a determination of response to chemotherapy. This is done by way of a combination of physical examination and imaging.

Treatment

Surgery

Patients with inflammatory breast cancer are managed with systemic therapy (such as chemotherapy) before surgery. We have long known that surgery *alone* as the primary treatment for inflammatory breast cancer yields poor outcomes. Surgery is used if the cancer has responded well.

What type of surgery?

Surgery is used to treat inflammatory breast cancer, and typically involves complete removal of the breast (mastectomy) and dissection of underarm nodes. Unfortunately, breast-preserving surgery for inflammatory breast cancer has resulted in poor cosmetic outcomes, and the available data suggests a higher risk of the cancer returning locally (breast/chest wall) as compared to a breast removal, or mastectomy.

The standard is to perform a breast removal (mastectomy) with an **axillary node dissection.** The use of the less invasive sentinel node procedure, wherein only one or two underarm nodes might be removed, does *not* represent an accurate way of assessing the response in the nodes to chemotherapy.

Can I have breast reconstruction?

If you have had a modified radical mastectomy (with removal of the breast and an axillary dissection of the nodes in the lower/mid-underarm area, known as a level I/II dissection), *delayed* reconstruction may be an option for you. We prefer that the reconstruction not be immediate, as it may compromise the radiation therapy that is given after the breast removal.

I did not respond to chemotherapy. What's next?

Some patients do not respond to systemic therapy given before surgery. For these patients, a mastectomy is typically not done; rather you may have additional chemotherapy and/or radiation therapy. If you then respond, a mastectomy is offered. Second line chemotherapy may include drugs such as carboplatin, vinorelbine, and capecitabine (Xeloda, an oral chemotherapy).

Treatment

Radiation therapy

Following mastectomy, you will very likely proceed to radiation therapy. This form of high-energy X-rays is designed to target cancer cells that may be in the chest wall and/or regional nodes. The timing and dose of your radiotherapy depends on how well your cancer responded to chemotherapy.

Radiation therapy targets include the chest wall (including the mastectomy scar) and regional nodes. The latter include the axillary (underarm) and paraclavicular (above and below the collarbone) nodes. Selected patients may also have internal mammary nodes (next to the breast bone or sternum) treated.

Here are seven key points about radiaton therapy, taken from a wonderful resource (www.breastcancer.org):

- Radiation is a targeted therapy designed to kill cancer cells that may still exist after surgery.
- The actual delivery of radiation therapy is painless. but radiation itself may cause some discomfort over time.
- External radiation treatment, the most common kind of radiation therapy, does not make you radioactive.
- Treatment is usually given 5 days a week for up to 7 weeks. The daily appointments usually take about 20 minutes.
- Radiation will not make you lose your scalp hair, unless it is given to your head.
- In the targeted areas, your skin can turn pink, red, or tan, and may be sensitive and irritated. Creams and other medicines may provide relief.
- During your treatment course, you may feel tired. This feeling can last for a several weeks -- even months -- after treatment ends. Most radiation side effects are temporary.
- Radiation therapy can significantly decrease the risk of cancer returning.

Treatment

Endocrine therapy: Targeting estrogen

If your cancer "feeds" on the hormones estrogen and/or progesterone, it is considered hormone receptor positive. Endocrine therapy will be offered to you after completion of chemotherapy. Several meta-analyses (looking at a collection of studies) have shown **endocrine therapy consistently improves survival odds** for those with invasive breast cancer that is estrogen receptor (ER) and/or progesterone receptor (PR) positive.

The approaches used include:

• **Tamoxifen**, the selective estrogen receptor modulator (SERM). It is a pill taken on a daily basis, typically for at least five years. For breast cancer in general, it can drop the probability of death from breast cancer by nearly a third.

• **Aromastase inhibitors,** which block the conversion of androgens ("male hormones") to estrogens in the adrenal glands (on top of your kidneys) and body fat. Examples of these drugs include anastrazole, letrozole, and exemestane. These pills cannot be used if you are still menstruating. When compared with tamoxifen, AIs result in a greater reduction in recurrence rates, and a lower probability of death from breast cancer.

• **Ovarian suppression** or ablation, which inhibits the production of estrogen from the ovaries (for pre-menopausal women). This can be accomplished in a number of ways, including the removal of the ovaries surgically, or through shots that shut down the production of estrogen in the ovaries.

Some patients will take tamoxifen, others an aromatase inhibitor, and still others tamoxifen followed by an AI. Total treatment duration is usually a minimum of five years.

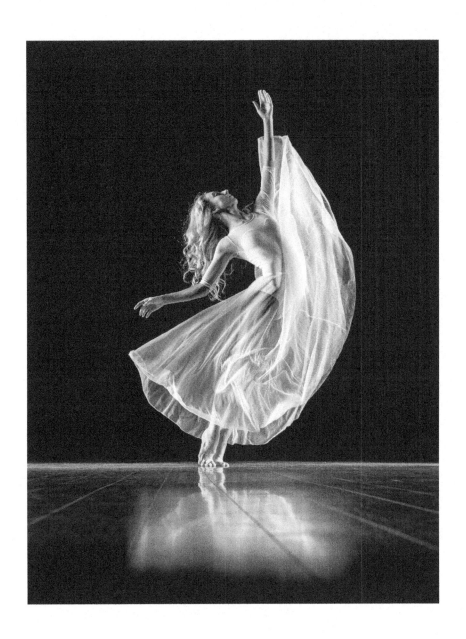

MANAGEMENT

CHEMO: DETAILS

Inflammatory

Management: Chemotherapy details

How

- Chemotherapy is most commonly injected into a vein. Less commonly, it may be given in pill form or injected into the muscle or fat tissue below the skin.

When

- Before breast removal: Neoadjuvant (*neo* - before; *adjuvant* - in addition to) chemotherapy is used for inflammatory breast cancer that has not spread to distant sites.

- Chemotherapy should begin within weeks of diagnosis. Please move with all due deliberate speed.

- Drugs are often given on a 14, 21, or 28-day cycle.

- Total treatment length varies, but often lasts from 3 to 6 months.

What

- Chemotherapy often works best with **combinations** of drugs. There are many chemotherapy regimens, and your medical oncologist and you will select one based on factors such as your age and health, cancer characteristics (including grade, HER2 status, and estrogen receptors), and stage.

- Some drug combinations are illustrated on the next page. For inflammatory breast cancer, a so-called **anthracycline (such as doxorubicin) plus a taxane (for example, taxol) is preferred** (National Comprehensive Cancer Network Guidelines, 1.2019). If HER2 is positive for overexpression, anti-HER2 drug(s) are added to chemotherapy.

Chemotherapy regimens

Chemo	Names
CMF	cyclophosphamide (Cytoxan), methotrexate (Rheumatrex), 5-fluorouracil (Adrucil)
CAF (FAC)	cyclophosphamide (Cytoxan), doxorubicin (Adriamycin), 5fluorouracil (Adrucil)
AC	doxorubicin (Adriamycin), cyclophosphamide (Cytoxan)
TAC	docetaxel (Taxotere), doxorubicin (Adriamycin), and cyclophosphamide (Cytoxan)
AC, T*	doxorubicin (Adriamycin) and cyclophosphamide (Cytoxan), followed by paclitaxel (Taxol) or docetaxel (Taxotere)
TC	docetaxel (Taxotere), cyclophosphamide (Cytoxan)

* for inflammatory breast cancer, the use of an anthracycline drug (such as doxorubicin) plus a taxane is *preferred* by the National Comprehensive Cancer Network (www.nccn.org).

Inflammatory

Management: HER-2 positive

Breast cancer is a group of diseases, with several biologic subtypes. One subtype is known as HER2-overexpressing. HER2/neu (human epidermal growth factor receptor 2) is a growth-promoting protein that sticks out of the cell surface like an antenna. About 20 percent of breast cancers will have overexpression of the oncogene, and are called HER2-positive. At diagnosis, your cancer should be checked to see if you have higher levels than normal levels (overexpression) of HER2. For this very aggressive subtype of breast cancer, we have powerful treatment tools, including chemotherapy combined with drugs (such as trastazumab (Herceptin)) that target the HER2 pathway.

What qualifies as HER2 positive?

Your cancer (biopsy and/or surgical material) is tested for HER2 overexpression, typically by one of these tests:

- Immunohistochemistry (IHC) test: Score of 3+ (the scale is 0 to 3)*

- Fluorescent *in situ* hybridization (FISH)

Herceptin-based treatment: Who needs it?

The clinical trials that established the benefit of following surgery with Herceptin-containing systemic therapy limited eligibility to women with lymph node involvement by cancer or those without such involvement, but thought to be at high risk for recurrence. This latter group included women with primary cancers in excess of 1 cm in size. Still, there is lower level evidence to suggest that there may be significant benefit from Herceptin with chemotherapy for patients with smaller primary cancers.

---

* If the result is 0 or 1+, the cancer is HER2-negative (and will not respont to treatment with drugs that target HER2); if the result is 2+, the HER2 status is not clear ("equivocal"), and we need to do a FISH test to try to get an answer.

Background

In 1996, the US Food and Drug Adminstration (FDA) approved Herceptin as part of a treatment regimen containing doxorubicin, cyclophosphamide and paclitaxel chemotherapy as adjuvant treatment of patients with HER2-positive, node-positive breast cancer. The history of this revolutionary drug, and the critical role played by leaders such as Dr. Dennis Slamon, are detailed in Robert Bazell's book *Her-2: The Making of Herceptin, a Revolutionary Treatment for Breast Cancer.* The book is a medical thriller, and I think is well-worth the read. For those who prefer film, check out Living Proof with Harry Connick Jr.

The evidence

Several large clinical trials have demonstrated the effectiveness of chemotherapy plus Herceptin (trastazumab) for breast cancer in general. The approaches may be conveniently divided into ones that contain a type of chemotherapy known as anthracyclines (Adriamycin/doxorubicin is an example), and the non-anthracycline ones. Here are two landmark trials that established Herceptin as a breakthrough drug for those whose tumors overexpress HER-2.

	Who	What
NSABP B-31	HER-2 overexpressing *and* nodes involved with cancer	Chemotherapy (AC) x4 followed by paclitaxel chemotherapy, with or without Herceptin beginning with the first treatment of paclitaxel
NCCTG N-9831	HER-2 overexpressing *and* nodes involved *or* High risk*, but nodes uninvolved	Chemotherapy (AC) x4 followed by weekly paclitaxel (T) chemotherapy for 12 weeks (no Herceptin) *or* AC then T chemotherapy followed by Herceptin *or* AC then TH, followed by Herceptin

* Estrogen receptors negative and primary over 1 cm, node negative or estrogen receptors positive and primary over 2 cm

Researchers combined the two large studies looking at whether Herceptin (trastaszumab) improved outcomes. There were 4,045 patients included in the joint analysis, with a median follow-up of 3.9 years. The inclusion of Herceptin led to a near-halving of the risk of recurrence (hazard ratio 0.61), and a 39% reduction in the risk of death (hazard ratio 0.61). Researchers found similar benefits to Herceptin when they looked at the studies separately.

Downsides

There are some downsides. **Cardiac toxicity** was increased among patients treated with trastuzumab: The rates of serious congestive heart failure (CHF) or cardiac-related death in patients range from 0% (Fin-HER trial) to 4.1% (NSABP trial). In comparison, the NCCTG trial found the 3-year incidence of congestive heart failure or cardiac death to be 0.3% with no Herceptin, 2.8% with Herceptin following chemotherapy, and 3.3% in the Herceptin initially combined with paclitaxel chemotherapy groups. This points to the need for careful (and ongoing) monitoring for cardiac problems.

Tremendous benefits

A 2012 analysis of eight trials confirmed the benefits of adding trastazumab (Herceptin) to chemotherapy for patients with HER2- positive breast cancer:

- *Improvement in disease-free survival*

  Patients with HER2 overexpression were nearly half as likely to recur if they had Herceptin added to chemotherapy (hazard ratio for relapse 0.6). This benefit appears whether the Herceptin is given during and after chemotherapy or after chemotherapy alone. However, an improvement in overall survival was only seen with the first approach; sequential chemotherapy followed by Herceptin did not seem to provide the same benefit.

- *Improvement in overall survival*

  Patients who had Herceptin added to chemotherapy were one-third less likely to die than those who did not get Herceptin. While Herceptin for 6 months seemed to provide some benefit, the improvement was small and not statistically significant.

For patients with estrogen receptor-positive breast cancer, endocrine therapy is given *after* the chemotherapy portion of treatment is complete; the anti-estrogen drugs are given during (and after) the continuing Herceptin.

1/2

That's the approximate reduction in the risk
or recurrence with Herceptin combined with
chemotherapy, compared to chemotherapy alone.*

* for breast cancer in general; not inflammatory breast cancer specifically

Herceptin benefits long-lasting

The benefits of Herceptin appear to be long-lasting. The combined North Central Cancer Treatment Group and National Surgical Adjuvant Breast and Bowel Project studies published data at a median follow-up of 8.4 years. The addition of Herceptin led to a 37 percent improvement in overall survival, and a 40 percent improvement in disease-free survival.

How is Herceptin given?

Herceptin is administered by vein. In the period after chemotherapy, the Herceptin is given once every three weeks, and is generally well-tolerated. The infusion itself is typically much quicker than with chemotherapy.

How long will I be on Herceptin?

The 2012 meta-analysis (review of a collection of studies) supports the use of one year of Herceptin, rather than shorter periods of time. Here are some results from studies looking at various durations of Herceptin:

- *Herceptin: 1 versus 2 years*

  The Herceptin Adjuvant (HERA) trial included 5,090 women with HER2-positive breast cancer who had completed chemotherapy. They randomly assigned the patients to observation or Herceptin for one or two years. At eight year follow-up, there were no differences in disease-free or overall survival odds.

- *Herceptin: 6 versus 12 months*

  The Protocol for Herceptin as Adjuvant therapy with Reduced Exposure (PHARE) trial randomly assigned 3,380 women to 6 versus 12 months of Herceptin. At a median follow-up of 42.5 months, treatment for six months resulted in a lower two-year disease-free survival (91 percent, compared to 94 percent for one year of Herceptin). The shorter duration patients also were nearly 1.5-times more likely to die of the disease.

I had chemotherapy and Herceptin before surgery.

Herceptin typically continues for a cumulative one year. However, if you have residual cancer in the breast or regional nodes, recent data suggests a significant benefit from the addition of the drug trastuzumab emtansine (also known as ado-trastuzumab emtansine or Kadcyla) after surgery.

Special situations

Males

The Herceptin-based recommendations for those with HER2-overexpressing cancers are same as for women.

Pregnancy

Herceptin may not be used during pregnancy, as we don't have sufficient evidence to know if it is safe. It is also recommended not to breastfeed while on the drug. Selected patients may have *chemotherapy* after the first trimester.

Pre-existing heart issues

It is especially important to have close monitoring of cardiac function. Some potential factors that may increase your risk include: Age over 50, pre-existing cardiac problems, being overweight, and having high blood pressure.

An international clinical trial, known as NOAH, treated 230 patients with HER2-overexpressing locally advanced or inflammatory breast cancer. Researchers randomized patients to receive chemotherapy with or without a year of Herceptin. Here are the results at the 5 year mark:

	Chemo	**Chemo plus Herceptin**
Event-free survival*	43%	58%
Overall survival	63%	74%

* event defined as recurrence, progression, or death from any cause

Triple negative breast cancer: Into the future

Triple negative breast cancer (TNBC) does not have estrogen or progesterone receptors, nor does it have the overactive HER2 that drive the other subtypes of breast cancer. There are currently no drugs specifically designed to target triple negative breast cancer. Because TNBC does not have a primary driver that we have historically targeted, we have largely depended on treatments we have had for decades, including chemotherapy, surgery, and radiation therapy. Now, we finally have the first generation of therapies specifically targeting triple negative breast cancer. As is typical, these new drugs are first being tried in the setting of metastatic breast cancer (some early successes have been reported), and will be tried for earlier stage disease going forward. Let's look at one innovative approach.

Turning your immune system against the cancer

Researchers combined the new drug **atezolizumab** with a chemotherapy called nab-paclitaxel for patients with metastatic triple negative breast cancer. Atezolizumab is immunotherapy; it is a so-called PD-L1 inhibitor that counteracts a cancer's ability to hide itself from your immune system. Basically, your immune system's T cells have PD1 receptors that, when activated, turn off a T cell's cell-killing activity. Many cancers express PD-L1.

Atezolizumab blocks the ability of PD1 receptors to bind PD-L1, thus leaving T cells able to target tumor tissue. In other words, **when PD-L1 is blocked, cancer cells can no longer hide from T cells. This can lead to a greater anti-cancer effect than chemotherapy alone could do.** In a study of 24 patients, 42 percent responded to treatment, with the majority of responders achieving stable disease.

No endocrine (anti-estrogen) therapy

As triple negative breast cancers do not have estrogen receptors or progesterone receptors, anti-estrogen therapy (such as tamoxifen or an aromatase inhibitor) is *not* recommended.

1 Cancer cell presses the STOP button of the immune T cell to stop the attack.

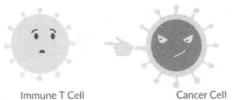

Immune T Cell   Cancer Cell

2 Checkpoint inhibitor blocks the STOP button, "taking the brakes off immune."

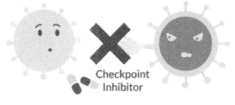

Checkpoint Inhibitor

3 Immune T cell is re-activated and can start attacking cancer cells.

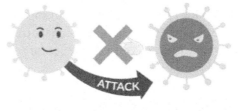

ATTACK

http://www.actgenomics.com/en/about

Inflammatory

Management: Chemotherapy

Selected side effects: Collateral damage

Chemotherapy can be associated with side effects. Most of the toxicity is temporary, and we have gotten better at managing side effects over the last several years. The specific side effects depend on the drug (or drug combination) that is used, and there is great individual variation in whether (and how) the side effects occur. Let's look at some of the more common side effects.

Nausea and vomiting

Your medical oncologist will discuss the use of drugs (anti-emetics) that can help reduce or prevent the nausea and vomiting that may occur during your course of chemotherapy. Many patients benefit from eating several small meals throughout the day.

"Chemo brain"

Chemotherapy can be associated with mental fogginess. In fact, a 2006 study from the Universty of Rochester showed that 82% of 595 individuals who received chemotherapy for cancer reported problems with memory and concentration. Brain imaging shows physiological evidence of so-called chemo brain: PET/CT imaging (to look at brain metabolism) shows that chemotherapy can induce changes in the brain that may affect concentration and memory. It is not uncommon to have these cognitive changes for 6 months after treatment.

Fatigue

Tiredness is among the most common side effects associated with chemotherapy. Physical activity may help improve your energy level. For many, the fatigue begins to improve weeks after completion of chemotherapy, although it may take 6 to 12 months for you to fully recover. Your supporters may benefit from your being very specific about how they can help you.

Mouth and throat sores

Chemotherapy preferentially affects rapidly growing cells. Given the cells in the mouth and throat turn over regularly, it is perhaps not surprising that some chemotherapy drugs can cause problems such as sores or dryness in the lips or mouth (including the tongue, gums, or roof or floor of mouth). Such drugs include (but are not limited to) capecitabine (Xeloda), fluorouracil, methotrexate, and doxorubicin.

Begin with a dental evaluation before you begin chemotherapy. During your course of chemotherapy, brushing your teeth (with a soft toothbrush) after each meal and before bedtime can be helpful, as can the use of toothpaste with baking soda and peroxide. Try to floss daily. If you smoke, stop. Ask your medical oncologist if you can eat a diet rich in fruits and vegetables. You may wish to avoid alcohol-containing mouthwashes.

Many patients who receive fluorouracil (5-FU) as a part of their chemotherapy find it helpful to swish ice chips or cold water in their mouths during the first 30 minutes of treatment: The cold appears to reduce the amount of drug that reaches your mouth. If you develop mouth sores, ask a care team member whether medications that coat the lining of your mouth might be appropriate for you. Some patients benefit from painkillers applied directly to the sore spot, but these can cause a bit of numbness (so be especially careful when brushing your teeth or eating).

Other helpful strategies may include avoidance of acidic, spicy, and hot (temperature) foods. Sharp and crunchy foods such as crackers, pretzels, and chips can be challenging for many. Alcohol should be avoided as well. On the positive side, try eating small meals more frequently (cutting food into small pieces and eating slowly). Consider using a straw to keep liquids away from mouth sores. Finally, try rinsing your mouth several times daily with a weak saltwater solution or a combination of baking soda and warm water.

Hair loss (alopecia)

During the course of chemotherapy, your hair may thin or fall out, depending on which drug(s) you receive. By hair, I also mean your eyebrows, eyelashes, and body. While the hair typically regrows shortly after completion of chemotherapy, the color and/or texture can change. Many patients will choose to cut their hair short beforehand, providing some degree of control. Others turn to mild shampoos and hair brushes, and use low heat when drying their hair.

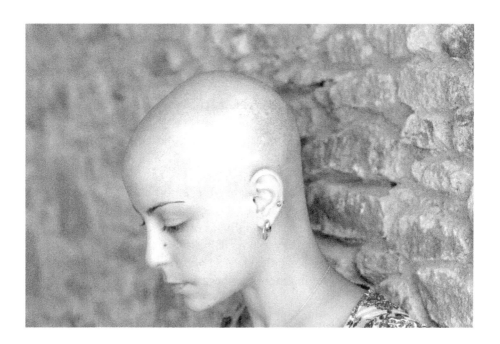

Hair loss

Within weeks after chemotherapy begins, many notice hair loss upon awakening, seeing it on their pillow. With brushing, they may see hair come out in clumps. This can be quite emotionally challenging. For many, wearing a wig, scarf, or cap can help them to feel more attractive. If you are told that your hair is likely to fall out, you can begin planning before chemotherapy begins.

- **Wigs:** If you decide to wear a wig, you may want to shop before treatment to match your hair color.

- **American Cancer Society** can direct women to places that can help them with wigs, and some ACS offices even provide offer wigs. Some insurance plans will help cover the cost of a wig.

- **Hats, turbans, and scarves** can also help hide hair loss, although some prefer to simply leave their heads uncovered. But, if you go bare-headed, don't forget the sunscreen for your scalp if you go outside.

- **Cutting your hair short** may ease the inconvenience of shedding lots of hair, and may make watching your hair fall out a bit less traumatic.

Scalp cooling for hair loss

Hair loss can be a devastating side effect of chemotherapy, but the recent US Food and Drug Administration (FDA) approval of the DigniCap Cooling System can improve the quality of life for many patients who receive chemotherapy. Historically, scalp cooling has not been available in the United States, in part because of concern that it wasn't effective at preventing hair loss, and because of concern about potential scalp metastases and thermal injury.

Scalp cooling devices lower the scalp temperature to prevent hair loss during chemotherapy. There are several methods to do this, but typically a hypothermia cap is connected to a computer-controlled cooling unit. A coolant circulates through channels in the cap, and sensors help keep the temperature in the appropriate range. The scalp cooling results in your blood vessels in the scalp constricting, reducing blood flow to the hair follicles while the chemotherapy is at its maximum. As a result, your hair follicles are less exposed to the drugs.

There are downsides. In the short term, many patients complain about a cold sensation ("brain freeze") and headache from the scalp cooling. Inflammation of the scalp and skin injuries are rare with device types that don't involve frozen caps. Fortunately, the data suggests that there is no increased risk of scalp metastases, at least at a average follow-up of 2.5 years in a USA study. In that study, the DigniCap system prevented hair loss in 66 percent of patients with breast cancer (compared to those who did not have the cap). Of note, the patients in the research had Stage I/II breast cancer and were receiving taxane-based chemotherapy. Those getting an anthracycline such as doxorubicin (Adriamycin) were excluded. While scalp cooling doesn't prevent you from losing some hair, it may reduce the volume of loss. Still, cost remains a significant issue in the United States, as you likely would have to pay out of pocket.

Other side effects

- Fever or infection
- Neutropenia or thrombocytopenia (low white blood cell or platelet levels)
- Dehydration or disturbances in blood chemistries
- Malnutrition
- Deep venous thrombosis of pulmonary embolism (clots that can spread to the lungs, sometimes becoming life-threatening)

Don't perm or color your hair during chemotherapy. Chemical treatments can enhance hair loss. Once your hair has begun to grow back (after completion of chemotherapy), you may perm or dye your hair.

Eyebrows and eyelashes

Some patients also feel upset about losing eyebrows and eyelashes. The American Cancer Society offers a program called "Look Good, Feel Better," that teaches women makeup techniques to improve their appearance during cancer treatment, including tips for eyebrows and eyelashes.

Nail weakness

Some chemotherapy drugs can cause damage to your fingernails and toenails. Your nails may become brittle and sore, and may even fall off. Fortunately, these problems are typically temporary. Still, if you develop nail inflammation or a rash that becomes open or is associated with a discharge, check in with your medical oncology team. The nail could be infected, and if needed treated with antibiotics. Those who do develop infection in separated nails may be recommended to soak their fingers or toes in a solution of white vinegar and water for 15 minutes every night. This can help kill bacteria, while drying out the area.

Infections

Chemotherapy may reduce the number of your infection-fighting white blood cells (WBCs), raising your infection risk. In this context, it is wise to wash your hands often and to stay away from others who are ill. Your physician should check your blood cell count before each treatment to make sure that you have enough white blood cells (and platelets and red blood cells) to give you chemotherapy. If you get a small cut or nick of the skin, please clean it immediately.

 It you have any signs of infection (such as a fever or shaking chills), please notify your doctor right away.

Skin

Chemotherapy often causes dry and irritated skin. You may wish to be proactive: One week before chemotherapy, begin measures to optimize your skin condition. Itching is common and can stem from multiple causes: the chemotherapy drug, a patient's naturally dry skin (particularly in people over 50), or as a symptom of the cancer itself. While many use over-the-counter hydrocortisone creams, they're often too weak to be effective, says Lacouture. Instead, doctors can treat itching with steroids or anesthetic medications applied to the skin. If itching interferes with sleep, oral medications might work.

Skin color changes can occur during chemotherapy, particularly with breast cancer treatment. The hands or face may be affected, making some feel self-conscious. If this happens bleaching creams and exfoliants with salicylic acid are available. Here is advice from Dr. Lacouture (Memorial Sloan-Kettering Cancer Center) who focuses on treating side effects related to the skin, hair and nails:

- Avoid long, hot showers or baths.
- Use gentle, fragrance-free soaps and laundry detergent.
- Use moisturizers, preferably creams or ointments rather than lotions (the thicker consistency is better at preventing skin dehydration). Apply the cream or ointment within 15 minutes of showering. Reapply at night, and moisturize your hands each time you wash them.
- If your skin is very dry and flaky, ammonium lactate cream can increase moisture. These are available by prescription and over-the-counter.
- Some chemotherapy drugs make skin more susceptible to sunburn. Use a sunscreen with at least an SPF 30, and make sure that it protects against both UVA and UVB rays. Protection against UVA requires ingredients such as zinc oxide, titanium dioxide, or avobenzone. Chemotherapy patients don't need to avoid the sun. Just be smart about sun exposure. Use a broad-brimmed hat, sun-protective clothing, and an SPF of 30 reapplied every two hours if you're outside, more if you are swimming or sweating.

Check with your doctor but, as long as there are no open sores on your skin, swimming is fine for chemo patients. However, hot tubs aren't a good idea. They can cause more blood flow to the skin, which can lead to greater blood flow to areas of inflammation. "There's no study that a hot tub will make it worse, but we tend to err on the cautious side," Dr. Lacouture offers.

Weight gain

Weight gain is commonly associated with chemotherapy for breast cancer. While the reasons are not entirely clear, chemotherapy can bring on menopause, which in turn can result in your gaining more body fat and losing lean muscle. Chemotherapy can also slow your metabolism, making it more challenging to keep weight off. Some women receive corticosteroids to help with chemotherapy-induced nausea and swelling, and these drugs can stimulate appetite, increase body fat, and result in loss of muscle mass in your upper arms and legs.

Try to eat well, and to get some physical activity: Aim for a minimum of the equivalent of a brisk walk for 30 minutes daily. If that is not achievable, try to do what you can.

Fluid retention

If steroids is a part of your chemotherapy program, you may develop water retention. Fluid retention can also promote weight gain. Fluid retention is usually only temporary. Here are some suggestions for management:

- Elevate your feet as often as possible
- Don't stand for long periods of time
- Try not to sit with your legs crossed
- Avoid tight clothing
- Reduce your salt intake
- Weigh yourself daily

Dehydration

Staying hydrated can help alleviate some of the symptoms associated with receiving chemotherapy.

Side effects

Nausea and vomiting: Additional tips

Here are some tips for managing nausea, courtesy of the wonderful website www.breastcancer.org:

- Eat small amounts of food all day long, so you don't feel full too quickly.

- Eat dry foods that are less likely to upset your stomach, like crackers, toast, and cereal.

- Stay away from greasy foods that might disagree with your stomach.

- Try ginger-based foods to help ease nausea. These include ginger ale, ginger tea, or crystallized ginger eaten as a snack.

- Sit up after eating -- lying down after meals may disrupt digestion.

- Rinse your mouth before and after meals to get rid of any bad tastes that may make you nauseated.

- Ask someone to cook for you or order take-out so you can avoid strong smells that may be unpleasant for you.

- Ask your doctor about anti-nausea medications that you can take before or along with your breast cancer treatment. There are also anti-nausea medications you can take with pain medications that nauseate you.

- Consider complementary and holistic techniques such as acupuncture, relaxation, and visualization to reduce nausea.

- Read tips on how to manage vomiting if nausea is making you sick.

Inflammatory

Special considerations

Fertility

If having children is important to you, talk to your care providers about your fertility options. Unfortunately, many caregivers do not provide sufficient information about the risk of infertility associated with various treatments for breast cancer, and many patients (who are concerned about fertility) are not referred to fertility specialists for counseling prior to cancer treatment. You should not become pregnant during treatment for inflammatory breast cancer.

The optimal time to begin fertility planning is at the same time as you are initiating breast cancer treatment planning. Alas, the very treatments designed to save or extend your life have varying probabilities of taking away your ability to conceive a child.

Chemotherapy and fertility
The majority of women under 35 years of age (and many over that age) resume menses within two years of finishing chemotherapy. Still, chemotherapy can result in the permanent loss of your menstrual cycles (periods). The risk, however, depends on the specific drugs administered. Risk increases with age: Women under 40 at the time of treatment are more likely than older women to have resumption of their periods after chemotherapy. The majority of women under 35 years old resume menses within two years of completing chemotherapy.

Tamoxifen ("anti-estrogen pills") and fertility
With tamoxifen, periods may return after treatment ends, although cycles may be irregular. Unfortunately, even if menstrual cycles return, treatment can shorten the time to have children. In addition, women on tamoxifen should not become pregnant, as the medicine has a risk of inducing birth defects. Typically, tamoxifen is taken for five or more years, and during this period the probability of natural fertility may decrease.

Storing embryos

What are some steps you may take before starting treatment in order to preserve fertility? One potential option is storing embryos. Here, eggs are collected over a number of menstrual cycles, fertilized and then frozen. After your treatment is complete, the embryos can be thawed and implanted into your uterus. Unfortunately, the collection of eggs can result in a delay to initiation of treatment, so check with your physician to see how long is acceptable. In addition, a sperm donor will be needed to fertilize the eggs before they are stored. Alternatively, unfertilized eggs (no sperm donor required) may also be frozen and stored. In the contemporary era, freezing unfertilized eggs may yield pregnancy rates similar to those achieved with fertilized eggs.

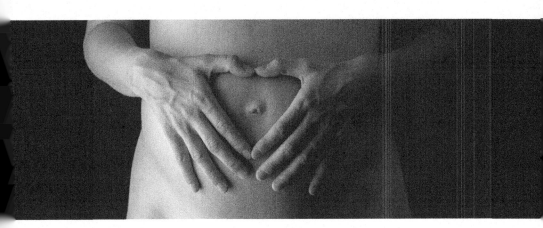

Protecting the ovaries

Chemotherapy acts on fast-growing cells. Still, there can be collateral damage to normal cells in your body, including the egg-containing ovaries. We have some drugs that can attempt to shut down the ovaries during chemotherapy, while potentially reducing the probability of early menopause. These include gosarelin (Zoladex), leuprolide (Lupron), and triptorelin. A meta-analysis (analysis of a collection of studies) found the use of such drugs to be associated with a higher rate of recovery of regular menses after 6 months (2.4-times as likely, as compared to those not on such drugs) and at least 12 months (1.85-times as likely) following the last chemotherapy cycle. In addition, these drugs were associated with a higher number of pregnancies (1.85-fold increase), although this outcome was not uniformly reported and rate of pregnancy was not the primary outcome in any of the trials.

MANAGEMENT
SURGERY: DETAILS

Invasive

Surgery

Two surgery types

- Lumpectomy - not generally done for inflammatory breast cancer
- Mastectomy (breast removal) - preferred for inflammatory breast cancer

For inflammatory breast cancer, a mastectomy is the standard surgery (after several cycles of chemotherapy are given), along with a dissection of axillary (underarm) lymph nodes, rather than the more limited sentinel lymph node removal. The latter is not generally recommended for IBC, as we have only limited data for the sentinel node approach. For those who do not respond to chemotherapy, management is individualized.

Surgery

You are taken to the anesthesia room, where a nurse inserts an intravenous (IV) line into your hand or arm, taping it into place. While many patients who have a lumpectomy have a local numbing anesthesia, some have general anesthesia. General anesthesia is typically used, especially given the removal/dissection of lymph nodes from the underarm area.

A total mastectomy (breast removal) is done, with a level I/II node removal (dissection of the nodes in the lower to middle portions of the underarm/axillary region). Skin-sparing mastectomy has not yet been demonstrated to be safe for those with inflammatory breast cancer. There is a need to remove currently or previously involved skin at the time of mastectomy.

Reconstruction

Immediate reconstruction is *not* recommended after mastectomy for inflammatory breast cancer, given the higher risk for recurrence, aggressive nature of the disease, and need to proceed expeditiously to postoperative radiation therapy.

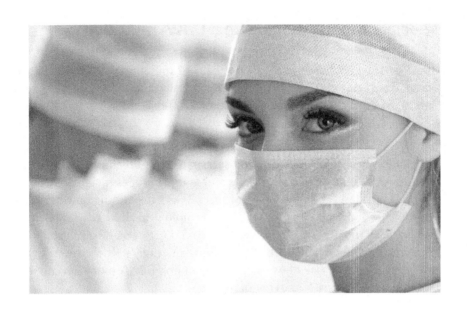

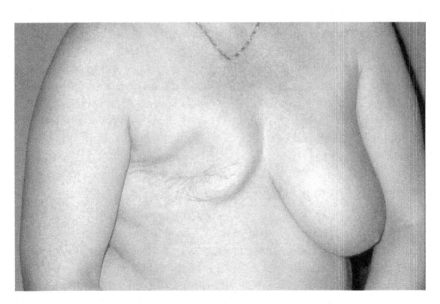

139

Genetics

A special note for those with a BRCA mutation

Many women with a harmful BRCA1 or BRCA2 mutation who develop breast cancer in one breast choose a bilateral (double) mastectomy, even if they would otherwise be candidates for keeping the opposite breast.

And the ovaries, too?

We do not have very effective tools for ovarian cancer screening. You may also wish to consider removing your ovaries and fallopian tubes in a procedure known as a bilateral salpingo-oophorectomy (BSO), depending on where you are in your life and whether you wish to have biological children. Some women choose to delay the procedure until age 40 to 45. I recommend a referral to a gynecologic oncologist for a discussion about this surgery. The surgery appears to not only reduce the risk of ovarian cancer among BRCA mutation carriers, but also decreases the risk of dying of the disease.

Other risk-reducing surgery?

Risk-reducing removal of the ovaries and fallopian tubes is the procedure of choice, with a removal of the uterus (hysterectomy) not routinely recommended. I am unaware of national guidelines pointing to the taking of the uterus, even though there may be a small increase in the incidence of uterus cancer among BRCA mutation carriers. There is controversy about removing only the fallopian tubes, for those who want to keep their ovaries for some time. Alas, we do not have high-level evidence from clinical trials to support this limited approach.

Hormone replacement (HRT)

Prior to using HRT to manage menopausal symptoms in BRCA carriers who have had a risk-reducing removal of their ovaries and fallopian tubes, there should be a shared decision-making process including counseling about non-hormonal options and our lack of high-level evidence regarding hormone replacement therapy for carriers of BRCA mutations. Similarly, we lack high-level evidence regarding the use of vaginal estrogen therapy for carriers.

Surgery: After

Management: Care after surgery

You will be moved to the recovery room, where care providers monitor your heart rate, blood pressure, and temperature. Most patients having a lumpectomy leave the same day, unless lymph nodes are removed. As you recover at home, you may need to:

• Take pain medication
Many patients have the prescription filled on their way home. While you may or may not need the pain medicine, it is wise to have it available.

• Take care of a bandage
Your surgeon or valued care team member should give you instructions. On occasion, the surgeon will ask you to wait until your first follow-up visit, at which time the bandage (dressing) may be removed.

• Stitches and staples
Stitches (sutures) are typically used, and dissolve over time. It is not rare to see the end of the stitch (suture) sticking out of the incision like a whisker. If this is the case, your surgeon can remove it. Staples are not common, but if used, they are removed during your first post-operative follow-up visit.

• Consider a good support or sports bra.
This may reduce movement that can cause pain. Many with larger breasts prefer to sleep on the side that has not been operated upon, sometimes with the healing breast supported by a pillow in front of them.

• Consider sponge baths until your doctor removes your drains and/or stitches (sutures)
Sponge baths may prove refreshing until your doctor gives you the okay for showers or baths.

MANAGEMENT
RADIATION: DETAILS

Treatment

Radiation therapy

Following mastectomy, radiation therapy is recommended for all patients with inflammatory breast cancer (following completion of any planned chemotherapy). Why radiation therapy? The chances of the cancer recurring in the lymph nodes or on the chest wall is high for individuals with inflammatory breast cancer. Radiation therapy can significantly reduce this risk. The radiation therapy fields are typically comprehensive, covering not only the chest wall, but the regional nodes in your axilla, around the collarbone, and (for some patients) next to the sternum or breast bone (internal mammary nodes).

While a survival benefit for radiation therapy has not been definitively proven, it is quite important as **radiation therapy can help optimize cancer control on the chest wall and in the regional lymph nodes.** Most patients receive approximately five weeks of daily radiation therapy (Monday through Friday), followed by a "boost" (over a week or so) to the mastectomy scar. In technical terms, we typically give 50.4 or 50 Gy (pronounced "gray") in 1.8 to 2 Gy fractions to the chest wall and regional nodes, followed by a 10 Gy (in five fractions) boost to the mastectomy.

An alternative radiation therapy dose scheme uses what we call accelerated hyperfraction. What we mean by this is that the treatment course is compressed, by giving two treatments daily (Monday through Friday, typically). While this approach may increase side effects, it may be appropriate for selected patients; for example, for those under 45 years of age; close or involved surgical margins; four or more nodes involved with cancer following chemotherapy; or a poor response to pre-surgery chemotherapy.

M.D. Anderson Cancer Center found twice-daily radiation therapy to 66 Gy led to improvements in chest wall/nodal control, disease free survival, and overall survival. The Memorial Sloan-Kettering Cancer Center reported similar local control rates without dose escalation, but using daily bolus (a material placed on the skin to optimize dose to it).

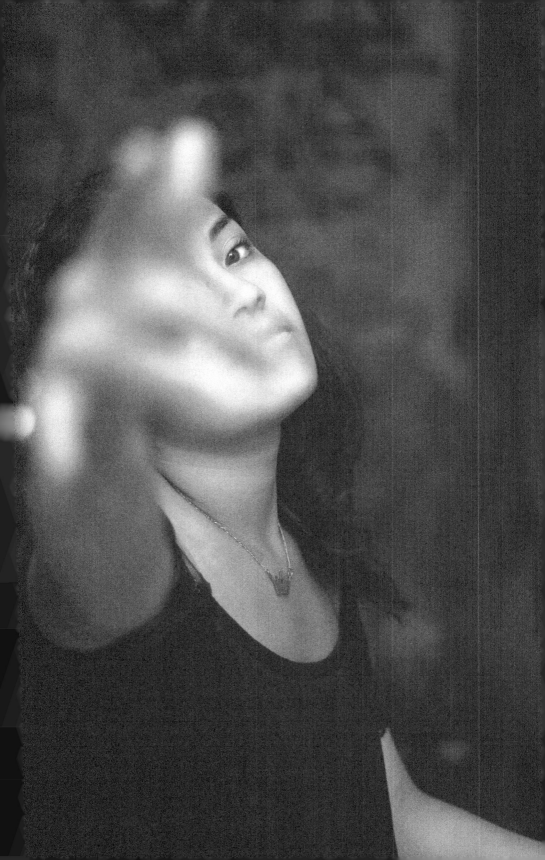

Management: Radiation after surgery

The challenge: Excess heart disease

Left breast or chest wall radiotherapy can deliver dose to the heart and coronary vessels, raising the risk of future cardiac events, including death. In an analysis of heart disease in a Nordic group of survivors of breast cancer, researchers found a significant excess risk associated with radiation therapy, a finding consistent with the risks seen in other radiotherapy-treated groups.

One potential solution: Respiratory gating

If radiation therapy hits the heart, it can potentially cause heart attack or even cardiovascular death. Today, we have innovative means to protect the heart. Respiratory gating software can be integrated into the radiation treatment plan. Your radiation oncologist can then define a physical window (like a baseball strike zone) and deliver radiation therapy only when the target is in this strike zone as you breath in and out. This technique can lead to the sparing of a greater amount of normal tissue such as the heart.

Example: Varian Real-time Position Management

This non-invasive, video-based approach allow clinicians to correlate target position in relation to your breathing cycle. Using an infrared tracking camera and a reflective marker, the sustem measures your respiratory patterns and displays them as a waveform. Your radiation oncologist then sets gating thresholds so that the radiation therapy beam turns off if your movement leaves you outside of preset limits.

Example: Elekta Versa HD system

Active Breathing Coordinator helps patients pause their breathing at a precisely indicated volume - a deep-inspiration breast-hold - which increases the distance between the tumor and critical structures, resulting in the ability to reduce doses to critical structures.

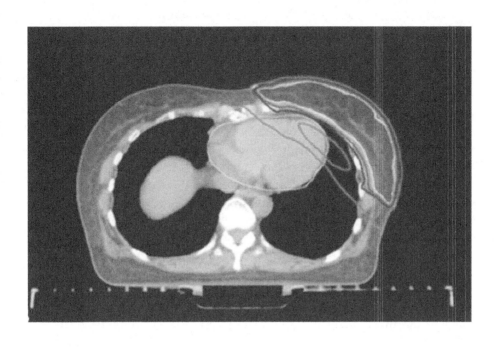

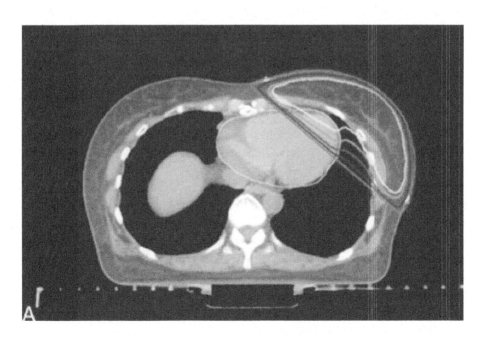

Short-term side effects

Whole breast radiation therapy may be associated with side effects, including breast skin fibrosis/scarring (4 percent), and decreased range of motion (1 percent). Mild generalized fatigue is common, often lasting for a month or two after completion of radiation therapy.

Longer-term side effects

• **Lymphedema:** Both surgery and radiation therapy can lead to early or delayed swelling of the breast, chest, or arm. Risks are highest among those who have a mastectomy with axillary node dissection followed by chest wall and axillary (underarm nodes) radiation therapy.

• **Nerve injury:** Uncommonly, RT can cause brachial plexopathy, damage to a nerve bundle at the top of your chest. This can cause weakness, or a tingling/burning sensation in the arm or hand. RT to the nodes around the collarbone may cause nerve injury in less than 1 percent of patients.

• **Lungs:** Radiation therapy to the breast region can result in lung inflammation (pneumonitis). Patients who have it may present with a persistent dry cough or shortness of breath. With today's techniques, pneumonitis is rare.

• **Heart:** Incidental radiation to the heart (as a part of treatment to the chest wall region for **left-sided cancers**) can result in a myriad of heart problems. These can include coronary artery disease, heart muscle injury, valve problems, and others. Technique matters greatly: Historic approaches often delivered relatively large doses to the heart or its vessels.

Once we recognized the radiation therapy side effects, we modified treatment techniques to substantially reduce heart irradiation. This is especially important for those who have received chemotherapy (or other drugs) that can damage the heart.

We have gotten better: In a study from the US Surveillance, Epidemiology, and End Results (SEER) database, the risk of death among those treated from 1973 to 1989 from ischemic heart disease was 13.1 versus 10.2 percent, when comparing left breast cancers to right ones. **For 1985 to 1989, the fifteen year death rates were not significantly different when comparing left and right side radiation therapy.** In our center, we use an innovative respiratory gating system, wherein the heart falls away from the target left chest wall, at which time the radiotherapy is delivered.

inspire

Management: Radiation therapy (RT) side effects

• **Musculoskeletal:** Breast and axillary surgery can cause reduced arm mobility. RT can worsen surgery-related pain and motor restriction in both the short- and long-term. Rib fractures from modern radiation therapy are uncommon, with a median time of about a year to its development.

• **Radiation therapy can uncommonly cause cancer,** including a 1 in 1000 risk of an aggressive angiosarcoma. The risk increases with dose, length of time after RT, and with younger age at the time of RT. We'll turn to other potential side effects of radiation therapy over the next couple of pages.

Leukemia

Rarely, radiation therapy can induce this blood cancer, or a condition known as myelodysplastic syndrome.

Lung cancer

The risk of lung cancer is higher among women who have had radiation therapy after a mastectomy as a part of treatment. The risk may not be increased for women who have had radiation therapy to the breast after a lumpectomy. The increased risk is first seen approximately ten years after radiation therapy, and can increase over time. The risk is higher for those who smoke cigarettes.

Sarcoma

Radiation therapy to the breast/chest wall region can increase your risk of a sarcoma of the blood vessels (angiosarcoma), bone (osteosarcoma), and other connective tissues in the radiation therapy volume. Fortunately, the risk if quite low.

Summary

Breast cancer treatment rarely causes cancer. The risk of a new primary non-breast cancer after breast cancer treatment is nicely illustrated by a review of 58,068 Dutch patients diagnosed with invasive breast cancer between 1989 and 2003. With a median follow-up of 5.4 years, here is what they discovered:

Radiation-induced cancer: Under 50 years old

Radiation therapy increased lung cancer risk 2.31-fold. Interestingly chemotherapy for this age group actually *decreased* second non-breast cancers (including colon and lung cancer) by a relative 22 percent.

Radiation-induced cancer: Over 50 years old

Radiation therapy increased the second non-breast cancer risk by a factor of 3.43. Chemotherapy raised the risks of melanoma, uterus cancer, and a form of leukemia known as AML.

We as caregivers should remain alert to the occurrence of second non-breast cancers. And you may reduce your risk with physical activity, a balanced diet, refraining from smoking, and optimizing your weight.

MANAGEMENT

ENDOCRINE: DETAILS

Invasive

Management: Endocrine therapy

Action Point

High-level evidence (including meta-analyses, or reviews of collections of research studies) shows endocrine ("anti-estrogen")
therapy improves survival among women with non-metastatic,
hormone receptor-positive (estrogen receptor and/or progesterone receptor positive) invasive breast cancer. There is consensus
that women who fit this profile should receive endocrine therapy.

Background

Some breast cancer cells use estrogen and/or progesterone ("female" hormones
produced in the body) to fuel their own growth. When these hormones attach
to proteins called hormone receptors, the cancer cells with these receptors
grow. All breast cancers are checked to see if they are estrogen receptor-positive (ER +) or ER -. The pathologist determines the receptor status by testing
the tumor tissue removed during a biopsy or surgery. Most breast cancers are
hormone receptor-positive. **Hormone (endocrine) therapies are only used to
treat hormone receptor-positive (ER+ and/or PR +) breast cancers.**

How do they work?

Endocrine therapies slow or stop the growth of hormone receptor-positive
tumors by preventing the cancer cells from getting the hormones they need to
grow. Some hormone therapies (for example, tamoxifen) attach to the receptor in, or on, the cancer cell, therefore blocking estrogen from attaching to the
receptor. An alternative approach lowers estrogen levels in the body, depriving
cancer cells of the estrogen they need to grow. The aromatase inhibitors are
examples of this second approach.

OESTROGEN **FUELS THE GROWTH AND DIVISION OF BREAST CANCER CELLS**

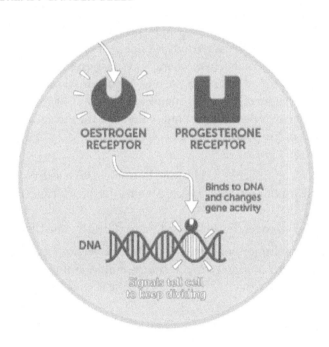

Naming

I prefer the terms endocrine therapy, or anti-estrogen treatment. Others use the somewhat confusing term "hormone therapy." The so-called hormone therapy used as a treatment for breast cancer is very different from that which is used as hormonal replacement therapy for women struggling with symptoms related to menopause.

Because the endocrine therapy approach can hinge on your menopausal status, we should first define menopause:

> **menopause** [men'-uh-pawz]. noun.
>
> The National Comprehensive Cancer Network (www.nccn.org) considers women 50 and older to be post-menopausal if there have been no menstrual periods for one year or more (in the absence of tamoxifen, chemotherapy, or ovarian suppression) and the estradiol blood level is in the post-menopausal range. Women are also considered to be postmenopausal if there have been have no menstrual cycles while on tamoxifen and the estradiol blood levels are in the postmenopausal range.

There are several approaches to blocking hormones such as estrogen from driving the growth of an estrogen receptor-positive breast cancer:

- Selective estrogen receptor modulator (SERM; tamoxifen)
- Aromatase inhibitors, which block the conversion of androgens ("male" hormone) to estrogens (for example, aromatase inhibitors such as anastrazole (Arimidex), letrozole (Femara), and exemestane.
- Reduction (or destruction) of ovary function

Examples of aromatase inhibitors include anastrazole (brand name Arimidex); letrozole (Femara); and exemestane (Aromasin). These drugs are only for women in menopause, as they block the creation of estrogen in the body fat and adrenal glands, but do not block estrogen production from the ovaries. Some women discontinue an aromatase inhibitor within the first five years. It is considered reasonable to then switch to tamoxifen after at least two years of the aromatase inhibitor drug have been completed. On the next page, we get some idea of the benefits of endocrine therapy for the general breast population (non-inflammatory breast cancer).

Aromatase inhibitor (AI) benefits
(not specific to inflammatory breast cancer)

	Aromatase inhibitors versus tamoxifen
AI (5 years) versus tamoxifen (5 years)	From years 0 to 1, the AI dropped recurrence by 1/3 (relative risk 0.64); from years 2 to 4, the relative risk dropped by 1/5. After 5 years, there was no further impact on recurrence.
Tamoxifen (5 years) versus tamoxifen for 2-3 years, followed by AI (total 5 years of endocrine therapy)	From years 2 to 4, the AI-containing group had recurrence drop by nearly 1/2 (relative risk 0.56); After 5 years, there was no further impact on recurrence. There appeared to be fewer deaths from breast cancer associated with the switch to an aromatase inhibitor.
AI (5 years) versus tamoxifen (2-3 years) followed by an AI (total 5 years of endocrine therapy)	From years 0 to 1, the AI lowered recurrence rates (relative risk 0.74) compared to tamoxifen. From years 2 to 4, there were similar recurrence risks. Finally, the use of the AI alone led to a trend towards reduced breast cancer mortality, but it did not reach statistical significance (relative risk 0.89).

AIs and premenopausal women

Aromatase inhibitors (AIs) don't normally work in pre-menopausal women because their ovaries are still making estrogen, and the drugs don't block estrogen in the ovaries. However, some pre-menopausal women may take an aromatase inhibitor when combined with ovarian suppression (for example, drugs* that shut down the ovarian function), which shuts down the ovaries. Indeed, some findings suggest ovarian suppression plus an aromatase inhibitor may reduce breast cancer recurrence better than ovarian suppression plus tamoxifen, although this question has not been asked specifically for those with inflammatory breast cancer. For non-IBC, this improvement is reflected in reductions in local, regional, and contralateral breast events and in distant recurrence chances.

* examples include leuprolide (Lupron) and goserelin (Zoladex); alternatively, the ovaries may be surgically removed.

Invasive

Management: Endocrine therapy

Action Point
For most women with estrogen- and/or progesterone receptor positive, postmenopausal breast cancer, an aromatase inhibitor pill is recommended, as it improves recurrence and survival outcomes compared with tamoxifen. While 5 years of an AI is standard, emerging evidence suggests 10 years is better (albeit with an increase in complication risks) for selected individuals.

Postmenopausal women

For most women with postmenopausal breast cancer, an aromatase inhibitor pill is offered. The so-called AIs are slightly better than tamoxifen at lowering recurrence and improving your survival odds. While the standard of care historically has been a 5-year course of an aromatase inhibitor, we have some 2016 data to suggest that 10 years might provide additional benefit (although with some increase in side effect risk).

Five years of aromatase inhibitor (AI) therapy either as up-front treatment or after 2-5 years of tamoxifen has become the standard of care for postmenopausal women with hormone receptor positive *early breast cancer*. The Canadian Cancer Trials Group MA.17R tested the benefit of extending an aromatase inhibitor for an additional five years using letrozole. Here are the results: 95 percent of the women in the 10 year letrozole group experienced disease-free survival, compared with 91 percent in the 5 year group. However, women who were treated with the drug for a total 10 years didn't live longer than those who were given a placebo in the study. Still, I think it is likely that a survival benefit will emerge in the data in coming years.

Some women may choose to begin with tamoxifen, with consideration of a switch to an aromatase inhibitor within the first five years. Alternatively, one may take 5 years of tamoxifen, and then swith to the AI for another 5 years.

Some women discontinue an aromatase inhibitor within the first five years. It is considered reasonable to then switch to tamoxifen after at least two years of the AI have been completed.

How long?

Approximately 70% of breast cancers are hormone receptor positive. The risk of recurrence among those in this population can persist for as long as 25 years or more after diagnosis. Five years of anti-estrogen (endocrine) therapy can reduce the risk of recurrence by about half, and mortality by nearly a third. Recently, we got data from the ATLAS trial showing extending tamoxifen therapy to 10 years reduced risk for breast cancer recurrence, as well as breast cancer-related death.

However, the optimal length of treatment with aromatase inhibitors such as anastrazole (Arimidex) and letrozole (Femara) - often used instead of, or after, tamoxifen to stop estrogen production in postmenopausal women - is controversial. In support of extended treatment, the MA.17R trial showed 10 years of letrozole reduced local recurrences and the development of cancer in the opposite breast, as compared to 5 years of the drug. On the other hand, the the difference in distant recurrence (metastases) was quite small.

Downsides

The use of aromatase inhibitor drugs is associated with an increased risk of adverse events, such as bone loss, fractures, bone and joint pain, hot flashes, and vaginal dryness. There are ways to reduce your chances for bone fracture and osteoporosis. Still, each individual and her clinicians will need to weigh the risks against the long-term projected benefits of extended anti-estrogen therapy beyond 5 years.

Invasive

Premenopausal women: Tamoxifen

Tamoxifen represents the gold standard of care. While historically the treatment lasted five years, extended tamoxifen to ten years should be considered for selected patients, for example those at higher risk of recurrence.

 An **aromatase inhibitor (AI)** pill is *not* appropriate as a single approach for women with intact ovarian function. This may include women who lose their menstrual cycles as a result of chemotherapy, as they may resume menstruating during follow-up.

Ovarian suppression: Only for those at higher risk

For patients at higher risk for recurrence (those under 35 and/or after those who received chemotherapy), consideration should be given to suppressing ovarian function (with injections) and adding an aromatase inhibitor (such as exemestane) instead of tamoxifen. Two clinical trials suggest that ovarian suppression with an aromatase inhibitor provides benefits behind those associated with tamoxifen, at least for higher risk women. Here are the patients who benefited from the more aggressive approach, at least according to a combined analysis of two clinical trials (SOFT and TEXT)*:

Patients under 35 years diagnosed with *early* (not inflammatory) breast cancer had a higher progression-free survival with ovarian suppression plus the aromatase inhibitor exemestane: Disease-free survival was 91% versus 87%, but there were no differences in overall survival odds. A subgroup analysis of the SOFT study suggested a benefit for the ovarian suppression-containing approach among patients treated with chemotherapy.

---

* Suppression of Ovarian Function Trial (SOFT) and Tamoxifen and Exemestane Trial (TEXT) - note that the study did not include those with inflammatory breast cancer.

The decision to incorporate ovarian suppression for those at high-risk is challenging as there can be significant side effects associated with this approach.

Side effects: Tamoxifen

A meta-analysis (analysis of a collection of studies) from the 2011 Early Breast Cancer Trialists' Collaborative Group compared tamoxifen for five years versus no endocrine therapy. Here are some (but not all) of the major side effects associated with tamoxifen:

- Deep venous thrombosis (blood clots, for example in your calf)
- Uterus cancer (limited to women over 55 years of age)
- Hot flashes
- Vaginal discharge
- Sexual dysfunction
- Menstrual irregularities
- Stroke (not statistically significant)

Hot flashes

Hot flashes are among the most common and troublesome toxicities of tamoxifen. They are thought due to a central nervous system anti-estrogen effect resulting in dysfunction of your body heat regulation system. Up to 80 percent of women on tamoxifen get hot flashes; for 30 percent they are severe.

There is variability among individuals in hot flash risk associated with tamoxifen. For example, premenopausal women are more likely to get them, compared to postmenopausal women. Genetics may play a role, too. In addition, some anti-depressant drugs known as SSRIs can decrease the conversion of tamoxifen to its most active byproduct (endoxiphen), influencing your chances of getting hot flashes. Examples include paroxetine and fluoxetine.

Blood clots

Tamoxifen can increase the risk of so-called thromboembolic disease, including pulmonary embolism (clots in the lung) and stroke. This elevated risk continues as long as you are on the drug. There may be additional risk when tamoxifen is added to chemotherapy, and the risk appears to rise if the tamoxifen is extended from 5 to 10 years.

Risk factors for developing clots in your veins include prior surgery, fracture, and immobilization. Your doctor may counsel you to discontinue the tamoxifen for several days prior to prolonged immobilization from planned surgery or travel.

An analysis of trials of tamoxifen from the Early Breast Cancer Trialists Collaborative Group demonstrated a non-significant excess of stroke deaths (3 extra per 1000 women during the first 15 years), but this risk was exactly balanced by a reduction in heart-related deaths (3 fewer per 1000 women).

Endometrial (uterus) cancer

Tamoxifen can raise the risk of both the common type of uterus cancer and a less common one known as uterine sarcoma. In the Early Breast Cancer Trialists Collaborative Group overview analysis of 20 trials, researchers found tamoxifen to be associated with a 2.4-fold increased risk of uterus cancer, but there was no increase in death linked to this increase in risk. The rate in the Breast Cancer Prevention Trial was 2.3 per 1,000 women per year, compared to 0.9 for the placebo group.

With long-term follow-up, we now know that tamoxifen results in a very small increase in the incidence of an uncommon cancer of the uterus: Uterine sarcoma (carcinosarcoma or malignant mixed Mullerian tumors) risk increases. The absolute risk of MMMT results in an additional 1.4 cases per 10,000 women per year.

Other tumors

While most individual clinical trials (including the largest one, the P-1 trial) looking at tamoxifen did *not* show an increases in non-uterine cancer, a meta-analysis of 16 randomized trials comparing tamoxifen with a placebo suggested a 1.3-fold increase in **gastrointestinal cancers.** We have some hints that tamoxifen may *lower* your risk of **ovarian cancer.** Still, we do not have high-level evidence to assert this with confidence.

Childbearing

Women of childbearing potential should use an effective means of contraception. Indeed, tamoxifen can induce ovulation. After stopping, check with your physician to see if you should be off the drug for a minimum of a few months to ensure that the drug has cleared your system.

Coronary heart disease

Among postmenopausal women, tamoxifen may not be associated with either a beneficial or adverse cardiovascular effect. The data are mixed. While tamoxifen can improve your lipid profile, it has *not* consistently been linked to a beneficial heart effect.

Eye problems

Tamoxifen has been found in some (but not all) studies to be linked to an increased risk of cataracts. The drug has been linked to dry eye, irritation, and retinal deposits that may cause macular edema. However, these side effects are uncommon. Your first line of defense? A baseline eye exam.

Other

Tamoxifen has been associated with vaginal discharge, menstrual irregularities, sexual dysfunction, and other problems.

Childbearing age

Women of childbearing potential should use effective contraception while on tamoxifen, as the drug can induce ovulation and also raise the risk of congenital abnormalities. After stopping tamoxifen, check with your physician to see if you should be off the drug for a minimum of a few months (before attempting to conceive a child) to ensure the drug has cleared out.

Side effects: Aromatase inhibitors (AIs)

- Musculoskeletal problems (bone pain, joint stiffness/achiness): Severe in about 1/3 patients, although the difference between placebo (inactive "fake" pill) versus aromatase inhibitors in randomized trials appears to be about 5 to 8 percent. Still, 10 to 20% will quit the AI because of these symptoms.
- Sexual dysfunction, pain, or dissatisfaction; hot flashes (35%)
- Reduced vaginal lubrication; reduced sexual interest
- Cognitive problems (forgetfulness, for example)
- Fatigue

Musculoskeletal (muscle/bone) syndrome

Aromatase inhibitors can be associated with joint pain or stiffness, and/or muscle or bone pain. For about a third of patients this symptom can be severe; on the other hand if we look at the difference between aromatase inhibitor and placebo (inert), there is a 5 to 8 percent difference. The bottom line? Musculoskeletal symptoms lead 10 to 20 percent of patients to stop the medicine.

The good news? There appears to be a dose-response relationship between exercise and symptom severity, at least according to the Hormones and Physical Exercise (HOPE) trial. The exercise regimen consisted of twice-weekly supervised resistance and strength training plus moderate aerobic exercise for 150 minutes per week. Other patients use non-steroidal anti-inflammatory drugs, but they have their own potential risks. Sometimes a switch to a different aromatase inhibitor can be beneficial. Some believe the antidepressant and nerve pain medication doxetine (Cymbalta) may provide some relief for patients for whom a switch to a different AI doesn't help. Finally, vitamin D might help. One study used vitamin D2, 50,000 IU capsule per week, and found it to be helpful. Such high-doses of vitamin D require close monitoring of blood levels.

Sexual dysfunction

Use of an aromatase inhibitor can result in vaginal symptoms and sexual dysfunction. Some patients describe reduced sexual interest, while others report diminished vaginal lubrication and/or pain with sex. Others mention orgasmic dysfunction and general dissatisfaction with their sex life.

Other side effects

Some women describe cognitive challenges associated with the use of an aromatase inhibitor. In fact, predictors of discontinuation of the drug by one year include:

- Fatigue
- Forgetfulness
- Poor sleep

Compared to tamoxifen, aromatase inhibitor use is linked with a *higher* risk of bone loss (osteoporosis), bone fractures, cardiovascular problems, and elevated cholesterol levels. On the positive side, aromatase inhibitor use can lead to a *lower* risk of venous thrombus (blood clots in your veins) and endometrial (uterus) cancer, at least as compared with tamoxifen.

Preferred aromatase inhibitor (AI)

The aromatase inhibitor seem to have equivalent effectiveness when used in the adjuvant setting (following surgery with curative intent).

Timing of aromatase inhibitor (AI)

Chemotherapy

For patients getting chemotherapy, it is generally recommended to sequence the chemotherapy before the endocrine therapy, although a meta-analysis from the Early Breast Cancer Trialists' Collaborative Group that compared concurrent with sequential treatment found similar drops in the risk for recurrence.

Radiation therapy

For women receiving radiotherapy after surgery, some clinicians have you start the aromatase inhibitor during radiation, while others wait until radiation therapy is complete. This author is unaware of data showing a difference in survival based on the timing of AI initiation relative to radiation therapy.

HER-2 positive

In the original clinical trials showing tremendous value for the addition of trastazumab (Herceptin) to chemotherapy for HER-2 overexpressing breast cancer, endocrine therapy was initiated (for hormone receptor positive cancers) once the chemotherapy portion of treatment was complete.

Non-compliance

One large study suggests that non-compliance with either tamoxifen or an aromatase inhibitor may increase your risk of death overall, although there appeared to be no influence on breast cancer-specific mortality. We join the National Comprehensive Cancer Network (NCCN) in encouraging compliance.

MANAGEMENT

DISTANT SPREAD

Metastases

Distant spread of cancer

> **metastasis [muh-TAS-tuh-sis]:** the development of secondary cancer growths at a distance from a primary site of cancer.

Distant spread of cancer is sometimes referred to as advanced, metastatic or stage IV (4) breast cancer. What all of these mean is that cancer has spread from the original site in the breast to more distant parts of the body. The most common sites of spread include the bones, liver, and lungs. The cancer can also spread to the brain or other body parts. In addition, metastatic cancer can affect one or more locations simultaneously. Spread to regional regions such as the axillary (underarm) nodes, paraclavicular (above or below the collarbone) nodes, or internal mammary nodes (next to the breast bone or sternum) may occur, but these are regional (and not distant) sites of spread.

  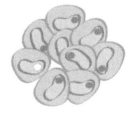

How does distant spread occcur?

Metastatic breast cancer develops when cells from the original cancer in the breast travel to distant parts of the body through the blood or lymphatic system. This new cancer is still known as breast cancer, even though it is in a different part of the body. Sometimes the cancer is present in distant sites at diagnoses, either macroscopically (we know about the metastases) or microscopically (our tests cannot show the distant spread, but it is present in small amounts). Alternatively, some cancer cells may survive treatment for what is initially non-metastatic cancer.

We have long believed that cancer metastasizes (spreads) when a single cancer cell escapes from the original tumor, travels through the bloodstream and sets up shop in distant organs. However, a growing body of evidence suggests that these bad actors don't travel alone; instead **cancer cells migrate through the body in cellular clusters, like gangs.** Roaming tumor clumps are led by a gang member that's fueled by a type of cellular kryptonite: a highly expressed protein called keratin 14. Understanding the molecular basis of collective dissemination may enable novel prognostics and therapies to improve patient outcomes.

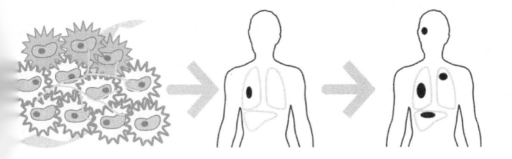

Metastases

Distant spread of cancer

Initial shock

You may be understandably devastated by the news that you have distant spread of cancer, or metastases. Some individuals experience anger, shock, or fear. It is understandable to have concerns about your future, and those of loved ones. Some women find a small amount of comfort with the knowledge that some women with metastases have lived for many years, experiencing long stretches of relative wellness.

No cure

While we do not yet have a cure for metastatic breast cancer, recent management advances mean that it may be controlled, often for years. For individuals who have a good response to treatment, the disease can sometimes be managed akin to a chronic illness: The cancer may be associated with periodic flares, but with extended times of wellness in-between these times of progression.

"How long do I have?"

Upon hearing that they have metastatic disease, many individuals first ask "How long do I have to live?" This is always difficult to answer, as every patient's experience is unique and individual and treatment factors can have large effects on survival. Whatever your individual situation, please know that treatments are continually improving and many women live for years.

Coping

- **Be informed**
  This can help you to understand your options for management.

- **Talk to a loved one**
  Let someone who cares about you know how you are feeling. This may help take off some of the burden of trying to keep a lid on everything.

- **Challenge unhelpful thought patterns**
  Check in with your care team about support resources such as social workers, mental health professionals, and other women in a similar situation) available to you. Many benefit from allowing themselves to be the center of their world, choosing with whom to interact and when to do so.

- **One step at a time**
  It may take a while to work out how you now want to live your life. Some women prefer to carry on with their usual daily routine, while others will want to completely alter their life. It can help to talk to those around you or to a health professional before making big changes. Try to take one step at a time and remember there is no need to rush into big decisions.

- **Share**
  Talking to others who have experienced secondary breast cancer may help –they may have an understanding of what you're going through. Every woman's needs are different. You can choose how much or how little information you need. Let your doctor know how you're feeling so s/he can help you manage any side effects early.

Metastases

Distant spread of cancer

Management overview

The type of treatment recommended to you will depend on the features of your metastatic breast cancer. This includes the areas in your body where your breast cancer has spread as well as the special features (pathology) of your cancer. Important factors include whether your breast cancer is hormone positive, or if it is HER2 positive, or if you have triple negative breast cancer.

Tools

While the management of metastatic breast cancer is highly individualized, commonly used treatment tools include::

- Chemotherapy
- Radiation therapy
- Targeted therapy (trastazumab (Herceptin) is an example)
- Endocrine ("anti-estrogen") therapy
- Surgery is less commonly used, although there are times when it may be recommended for you; for example to treat or prevent a bone fracture or to remove a single tumor in the brain.

Treatment options are tailored to you as an individual, but offer hope: While survival rates vary greatly from person to person, one study found that about 37 percent of women lived at least 3 years after diagnosis with metastatic breast cancer in general (not specific to inflammatory breast cancer). Some women may live 10 or more years beyond diagnosis. It is important to note that survival data are based on women diagnosed before some of the newer treatments for metastatic breast cancer were available. Modern treatments have improved survival for women diagnosed today.

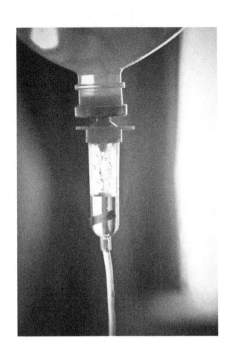

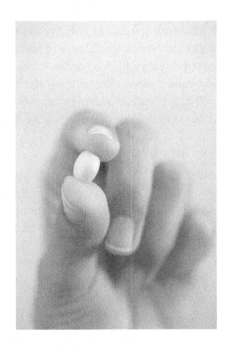

Metastases

Distant spread of cancer

Goals

Here are some of the primary goals of systemic treatment for the treatment of metastatic breast cancer:

- Survival prolongation
- Symptom relief (palliation)
- Quality of life maintenance

While the median survival is 18 to 24 months for metastatic breast cancer in general (not specific to IBC), many variables can affect the length (including cancer subtype, specific sites of metastatic disease, and volume of cancer). Some patients will even achieve long-term survival. Unfortunately, we do not have randomized clinical trials to prove that systemic therapy (such as chemotherapy, endocrine therapy and/or anti-HER2 strategies) prolong survival, when compared to best supportive care.

Role for repeat biopsy

Sometimes, the biology of a metastases is different from the primary breast cancer. This suggests a potential role for a repeat biopsy to reassess molecular markers such as estrogen receptors (ER), progesterone receptors (PR), and HER2 overexpression. This may be especially important when the primary cancer is negative for these markers, as a change to positive would likely modify treatment recommendations significantly.

How often do molecular markers such as ER, PR, and HER2 change? A pooled analysis of two prospective trials showed **discordance in ER, PR, and HER between the primary and recurrent cancer to be 13, 31, and 5.5 percent,** respectively. A separate study found similarly, with rates of discordance 13, 28, and 3 percent, respectively for ER, PR, and HER2.

Circulating tumor cells (CTCs) and tumor markers

Your doctor may (or may not) order blood tests to look for either tumor markers or cancer itself in the body. We can measure in-blood proteins that may be produced by your cancer; alternatively, circulating tumor cells that have broken away from the initial cancer and have moved into the bloodstream may be measured. Assessments of both protein markers and circulating tumor cells are made using a blood test. Here are some commonly used tumor markers:

- CA 15.3
- TRU-QUANT or CA 27.29
- CA125
- CEA (carcinoembryonic antigen)
- Circulating tumor cells (CellSearch test is approved by the US Food and Drug Adminstration)

While these tests may have some value, they are imperfect: If the tumor marker is great, it doesn't mean there is no cancer hiding; on the other hand, if the result is not good, it doesn't necessarily mean the cancer is progressing. The tests can be expensive, cause anxiety, and have *not* been associated with survival improvements for those with metastatic breast cancer. Still some find them helpful, at least for looking at trends over time.

Metastases

Distant spread of cancer

Prognosis

Here are some factors that can influence your prognosis if you have metastatic breast cancer:

- **Interval from initial therapy to relapse**
  A relapse-free interval of 2 or more years appears to be associated with a better prognosis, at least when compared to those with a shorter time to relapse.

- **Sites of metastases**
  If your metastases predominantly involves the bones, you may have prolonged progression-free and overall survival, as compared with those with liver and/or lung disease. Those with a a very high volume of disease in the liver, bone marrow replacement, or carcinomatous meningitis may have a poorer prognosis.

- **Cancer markers (ER, PR, HER2)**
  Hormone receptor (estrogen- and progesterone)-positive metastases are associated with a longer survival in general, when compared to ER/PR-negative disease. Those with HER2 overexpression or triple (ER/PR/HER2) negative breast cancer had a shorter medican survival, especially historically (when we did not have effective targeter therapies such as Herceptin).

- **Other**
  Other adverse prognostic factors include a poor performance status (your day-to-day level of activity), significant weight loss, and an elevation in your blood levels of serum lactic dehydrogenase (LDH).

Work-up

The National Comprehensive Cancer Network (NCCN) offers the following work-up for those with distant spread of cancer:

- History and physical exam

- CBC

- Liver function tests and alkaline phosphatase

- Chest diagnostic CT scan

- Abdominal ± pelvic diagnostic CT or MRI

- Brain MRI if neurologic symptoms

- Bone scan or sodium fluoride PET/CTh (if FDG PET/CT is performed and clearly indicates bone metastasis, on both the PET and CT components, bone scan or sodium fluoride PET/CT may not be needed).

- FDG PET/CT scan (optional, with PET/CT most helpful in situations where standard staging studies are unclear or suspicious)

- X-rays of symptomatic bones and long and weight-bearing bones abnormal on bone scan

- First recurrence of disease should be biopsied

- Determination of tumor ER/PR and HER2 status on metastatic site*

- Genetic counseling if you are at high risk for hereditary breast cancer

---

* In clinical situations where a biopsy cannot safely be obtained, but the clinical evidence is strongly supportive of recurrence, treatment may commence based on the ER/PR/HER2 status of the primary tumor.

Metastases

Distant spread of cancer

Bone involvement

Drugs

Your oncologist will likely recommend the use of drugs to reduce your risk of developing fractures, bone pain, and potential compression of your spinal cord. Examples include bisphosphonates, medicines used to prevent or treat osteoporosis. They work by limiting the activity of bone cells called osteoclasts. This then can help strengthen the bone and reduce the breakdown that leads to osteoporosis. But bisphosphonates have another important role: They may help prevent breast cancer from spreading to your bones by making it more challenging for cancer to grow there.

Reduction in bone problems, but no survival advantage

Drugs that target the breakdown of bone cells by metastatic cancer can lower the risk of bones breaking (fractures), reduce the chances that you will need radiation therapy to treat bone pain, and drop the chances you will develop levels of blood calcium that are too high. In addition, the use of these drugs can also reduce the chances you would develop cancer spread that puts your spinal cord in jeopardy (spinal cord compression). We have no evidence that any of these drugs lengthen your overall survival time.

Should I take one of these drugs?

They should be considered if you have bone metastasis, especially the lytic (hole punching) type and/or are in a weight-bearing bone, if you have an expected survival of 3 months or longer, and if your kidney function is adequate.

Selected drugs for bone metastases

- **Denosumab (Prolia; Xgeva)**
Under the skin (subcutaneous) injection every 4 weeks. Optimal duration remaining unknown.

- **Zoledronic acid (Reclast; Zometa)**
Monthly by vein for a year, then every 3 months for a total of up to two years. Longer may be better, but we lack high level evidence. These drugs should be accompanied by calcium (1200 to 1500 mg daily, in divided doses) and vitamin D (400 to 800 IU daily).

- **Pamidronate** (given by vein)
Monthly for a year, then every 3 months for a total of up to two years. Longer may be better, but we lack high level evidence. This medication is given by slow injection into a vein for at least 2 hours, but up to 24 hours, or as directed by your doctor. Pamidronate is generally accompanied by calcium (1200 to 1500 mg daily, in divided doses) and vitamin D (400 to 800 IU daily).

- **Ibandonate (Boniva):** Pill or by vein

- **Clodronate (Bonefos):** Pill

Zoledronic acid and pamidronate should be accompanied by calcium (1200 to 1500 mg daily) and vitamin D (400 to 800 IU daily). Bisphosphonates are typically given in addition to chemotherapy or endocrine therapy. Zoledronic acid may be superior to pamidronate for those with lytic bone metastasis. Finally, a 2012 meta-analysis found that the newer drug **denosumab was better than placebo, zoledronic acid and pamidronate** in reducing the risk of fractures.

Improved recurrence risk (for postmenopausal women)

Early research results were mixed on whether bisphosphonates help reduce recurrence risk. More recent data suggests that these drugs do reduce the risk of relapse, but only among postmenopausal women (or women who have been made postmenopausal through ovarian suppression).

Metastases

Distant spread of cancer

Bone involvement

Is one bisphosphanate better than the others? No.

A randomized trial looked at Bonefos, Boniva, and zoledronic acid. After 5.4 years of follow-up, 88% of the women were living and had not had a recurrence. This rate was the same no matter which bisphosphonate the women got. Looking at the individual cancer subtypes, there appeared to be similar benefits among the bisphosphonate drugs. Finally, the 5-year overall survival rate was 93%, with no survival differences seen when comparing the drugs.

Despite differences in the types of side effects, the overall severity of toxicity differed little when comparing the treatments. Patients generally prefer the oral drugs.

Side effects (toxicity): Collateral damage

While I will not discuss all of the potential side effects of these drugs, there are some that I want to review. Some individuals on bisphosphonate drugs or denosumab will develop bone, muscle, or joint pain. Let you health care provider know right away if you develop any of these. Some individuals who take bisphosphonates require an increase in vitamin D and calcium intake. If you develop muscle twitching or an increase in your level of anxiety, ask your care provider if you need to take vitamin D and calcium supplements.

 A rare, but serious complication is **jaw bone breakdown** (osteonecrosis). it is important to have a full dental exam before starting treatment and to talk with your oncologist before getting any dental procedure while on bisphosphonates or denosumab.

Bisphosphonate drugs may irritate your esophagus. When taking these pills, follow the directions carefully. They should be taken on an empty stomach with plenty of plain water while sitting or standing. After taking a bisphosphonate, please remain upright for at least 30 minutes and avoid eating, drinking or taking other medicines during this time. Be careful with the use of antacids.

Metastases

Distant spread of cancer

Bone involvement

Is there a potential role for surgery for bone metastases?

If you have a leg or arm that is very weakened by bone metastases, you may need an orthopedic surgeon to place a metal rod in the bone. This intervention can drop the chances of the bone breaking; if your bone has already fractured, you will likely need surgical stabilization. Several weeks later, a short course of radiation therapy is typically given to destroy cancer in that region. If the radiation takes out the cancer in that zone, the bone has a shot at rebuilding.

And if the cancer is causing destruction in my spine?

While not commonly needed, some patients have surgery for cancer spread to the spine. Other interventions may include the injection of bone cement into cracks (vertebroplasty). Kyphoplasty involves the insertion of a balloon to first widen the space inside the crack before the bone cement is injected. Such interventions are then usually followed by a short course of radiation therapy.

My blood calcium level is much too high. What are my options?

Your doctor offers that you have hypercalcemia, a condition in which you have too much calcium in your blood. Sometimes the cancer can cause it; in other cases, the cancer's effects on the bone can allow calcium to slip out into the bloodstream. Even some cancer treatment can result in an elevation of your calcium levels.

Unfortunately, having too much calcium can be a major problem. Potential interventions including: 1) giving you extra fluids; or 2) the use of drugs that reduce the calcium coming out of the bone into the bloodstream. Examples of such drugs include pamidronate/pamidronic acid (Aredia), zoledronic acid (Zometa; Reclast), and denosumab (Xgeva).

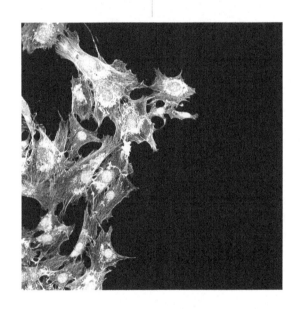

Metastases

Distant spread of cancer

Bone involvement

Is there a potential role for radiation therapy (RT) for bone metastases?

Yes, radiation therapy is the most common local treatment for cancer spread to the bone, and **RT can be especially effective for pain relief.** Radiation therapy can also lower the risk of breaking a bone in areas that may be weakened from cancer. In essence, high-energy X-rays can destroy cancer cells in the local area, permitting the bones to have a chance to rebuild. As we discussed in the previous page, surgery is sometimes offered before radiation therapy, particularly if a leg or arm is seriously weakened.

Radiation therapy uses high-energy X-rays (or particles, far less commonly) to try to destroy cancer cells. We typically aim a radiation beam to the target, using a machine located outside your body. RT is often given in either one large dose or over 5 to 10 days (Monday through Friday typically). The one large treatment approach is convenient, and offers a similar chance for pain relief. On the other hand, the longer course is associated with a slightly lower chance of your needing re-treatment to the same area, as described below.

Only slightly better long-term control with multiple treatments

The American Society for Radiation Oncology (ASTRO) Guideline statement is clear: Multiple randomized trials have shown pain relief equivalency for dosing schema including 30 Gy in 10 fractions (a fraction is a single treatment), 24 Gy in 6 fractions, 20 Gy in 5 fractions, and a single 8 Gy fraction for patients with previously un-irradiated painful bone metastases. Fractionated treatment courses are associated with an 8% re-treatment to the same anatomic site due to recurrent pain versus 20% after a single fraction, while the single fraction treatment approach optimizes patient and caregiver convenience.

184

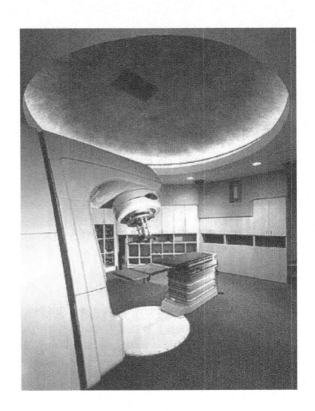

Stereotactic body radiation therapy (SBRT)

Stereotactic body radiation therapy (also known as stereotactic ablative radiation therapy or SABR) is a special form of external beam radiation therapy that gives large doses of radiation therapy for only one (or a few) days. Several X-ray beams are aimed at the cancer target from different angles. You do not feel anything during the delivery of the radiation therapy.

Side effects (toxicity): Collateral damage

Mild to moderate general fatigue is commonly associated with the receipt of radiation therapy, and it may last for a month or two. Other potential side effects are limited to the volume being hit by the radiation therapy. For example if we need to treat you cervical spine (neck), you may get a sore throat. If we target bones such as the ribs, arms, or legs, many individuals experience no side effects, other than a bit of general tiredness.

Metastases

Distant spread of cancer

Spinal cord compression: An emergency

Once diagnosed, spinal cord compression is a medical emergency. Spinal cord compression is a terrible complication of cancer spread to the spine. Many patients experience motor weakness and loss of sensation, and may even have bladder dysfunction. If it is not managed appropriately, the neurologic problems can progress rapidly to paralysis. If your care provider suspects you may have a compression, you will likely proceed immediately to an MRI imaging study of the spine.

Surgery: Suddenly Can't Walk?

You may be a candidate for surgery if you have a life expectancy of at least 3 months. The surgeon may approach the spine from the front, back, or a combination of the two (depending on the exact location of the problem). Surgery followed by a short course of radiation therapy can be quite effective in relieving the spinal cord compression and its associated symptoms. Here are the results of the only randomized trial addressing whether surgery plus radiation therapy (RT) is better than radiation therapy alone for those who could not walk, with the trial including several types of cancer:

	Surgery + RT	Radiation therapy
Regained walking	84%	57%
Kept walking	122 days	13 days

The study excluded patients with neurologic deficits for more than 24 hours, multiple spinal tumors, and prior radiation therapy. In addition, the in-hospital death rate was nearly 6 percent, and the complication rate was 22 percent.

186

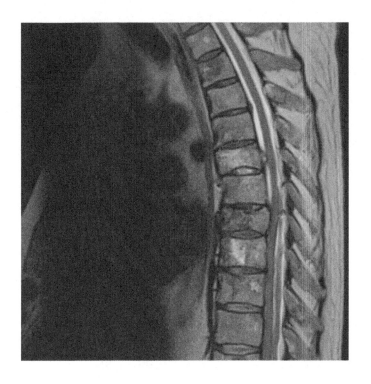

Spinal cord compression: Radiation therapy

Radiation therapy has long played a central role in the management of spinal cord compression. In the modern era, surgery may be used (particularly if you cannot walk), with radiation therapy offered thereafter. In order to allow for healing, we generally wait one to three weeks after the surgery before irradiating patients.

Radiation therapy can be quite effective especially for breast cancer. In one study using radiation therapy (without surgery), 70 percent of patients who could not walk regained the ability to ambulate, and the majority experienced pain relief. A typical course spans two weeks (10 treatments, with appointment times on the order of 15 to 20 minutes).

Metastases

Distant spread of cancer

Systemic treatment

Management of metastatic breast cancer is individualized, taking into account you tumor biology, clinical factors, and your goals. In general, those with only one site of cancer spread may benefit from an intense approach to controlling that lesion added to systemic treatment (such as with chemotherapy or anti-estrogen drugs).

Goals

- Survival prolongation
- Symptom relief (palliation)
- Maintenance or improvement of quality of life

Selecting: Anti-estrogen drugs versus chemotherapy

Many doctors believe that chemotherapy is associated with a higher probability of cancer response for those with hormone receptor-positive breast cancer (especially for those with cancer in organs such as the liver and lung), as compared with anti-estrogen (endocrine) therapy. We actually don't have recent high-level evidence to conclusively confirm that belief.

An historic meta-analysis (collection of studies) looked at several studies, all published before 1995. The researchers found higher response rates (by a factor of 1.25) with chemotherapy. Still, there were no differences in survival length, when comparing the two management approaches to one another. Over the next several pages, we will look at the various systemic therapy approaches for metastatic (secondary) breast cancer.

Management: Drugs

Prior endocrine therapy within one year

Premenopausal   Ovarian removal or suppression, plus endocrine therapy (with or without a drug designed to help overcome cell resistance that has developed to endocrine therapy; examples are so-called CDK4/6 or mTOR inhibitors) as for postmenopausal women.

Postmenopausal   Consider a different endocrine therapy (with or without a drug designed to help overcome cell resistance to endocrine therapy; examples are so-called CDK4/6 or mTOR inhibitors) as for postmenopausal women.

Visceral crisis   Consider initial chemotherapy if disease in organs such as the liver or lungs is particularly threatening.

No prior endocrine therapy within one year

Premenopausal   Ovarian removal or suppression, plus endocrine therapy (with or without a drug designed to help overcome cell resistance that has developed to endocrine therapy; examples are so-called CDK4/6 or mTOR inhibitors) as for postmenopausal women.

Postmenopausal   Options include aromatase inhibitor (or other) drugs or other endocrine approaches, such as a CDK 4/6 inhibitors with an aromatase inhibitor or fulvestrant.

Management: Drugs

CDK 4/6 kinase inhibitors

Palbociclib (Ibrance) is a prescription medicine used to treat hormone receptor-positive, human epidermal growth factor receptor 2-negative (HER2-) breast cancer that has spread to other parts of the body (metastatic) in combination with:

- an aromatase inhibitor as the first hormonal based therapy in women who have gone through menopause, or
- fulvestrant in women with disease progression following hormonal therapy.

How

Estrogen and hormone receptors contribute to the growth of certain breast cancers. In hormone receptor positive, HER2- metastatic breast cancer, the presence of estrogen and hormone receptors can cause an overactive signaling of proteins within the nucleus (center) of the cell that tells the cell to grow and divide.

Two of these proteins are called CDK 4 and CDK 6. The increased activity of these proteins inside the nucleus causes a loss of cell cycle control, which causes cells to grow and divide too fast. Palbociclib is a highly selective inhibitor of CDK 4/6 kinase activity. A randomized, multicenter trial evaluated the safety and efficacy of palbociclib in combination with letrozole versus letrozole alone as first-line treatment for patients with advanced estrogen receptor-positive, HER2-negative metastatic breast cancer.

Median progression-free survival was double with the combination regimen compared to letrozole alone (20.2 months versus 10.2 months). Significant side effects reported at a higher incidence in the palbociclib plus letrozole group included drops in a type of white blood cells (neutropenia - 54% vs. 1%) and white blood cells overall (19% vs. 0%). Based on this study, the US Food and Drug Administration approved palbociclib as initial endocrine-based therapy for metastatic disease.

The phase III trial (PALOMA-3) compared the combination of palbociclib and the endocrine therapy fulvestrant to fulvestrant in pre- or post-menopausal hormone receptor-positive, HER2-negative advanced breast cancer patients, whose disease had progressed on prior endocrine therapy. Women who had not completed menopause received a shot (goserelin) to shut down the function of their ovaries.

The median progression-free survival was 9.2 months for the combination compared to 3.8 months for fulvestrant with similar discontinuation rates because of adverse effects (2.6% and 1.7%, respectively).

CDK 4/6 kinase inhibitors: Side effects

Serious

• **Low white blood cell counts (neutropenia) are very common** when taking palbociclib (Ibrance) and may cause serious infections that can lead to death.
Your healthcare team should check your white blood cell counts before and during treatment.

• If you develop low white blood cell counts during management with palbociclib, your doctor may stop your treatment, decrease your dose, or may tell you to wait to begin your treatment cycle. Tell your doctor right away if you have signs and symptoms of low white blood cell counts or infections such as fever and chills.

Common

• **In addition to low white blood cell counts (neutropenia), low red blood cell counts and low platelet counts are common** with palbociclib. Call your healthcare team right away if you feel dizzy or weak, notice that you bleed or bruise more easily, or experience shortness of breath or nosebleeds while on treatment.

• Other common side effects include (but are not limited to) infections, tiredness, nausea, sore mouth, abnormalities in liver blood tests, diarrhea, hair thinning or hair loss, vomiting, rash, and loss of appetite.

Management: Drugs

MTOR inhibitors

MTOR inhibitors are drugs that help reverse the resistance your cancer cells may develop to endocrine therapy. The development of such resistance among women taking endocrine therapy for hormone receptor-positive breast cancer is common.

Resistance

One mechanism of resistance to endocrine therapy is activation of the a growth-triggering pathway known as the mammalian target of rapamycin (mTOR) signal transduction pathway. Can we inhibit this mTOR pathway to regain the cancer-slowing properties of endocrine therapy? The answer is yes.

Research findings

Several randomized studies have investigated the use of aromatase inhibition in combination with inhibitors of the mTOR pathway. One such trial looked at postmenopausal women with metastatic (advanced), hormone receptor positive breast cancer who had not received prior endocrine therapy for their metastases. Researchers randomized patients to receive letrozole (Femara), with or without the mTOR inhibitor temsirolimus. The study was negative, with no differences in progression free survival seen.

On the other hand, the so-called BOLERO-2 trial had positive results. Once again, postmenopausal women with hormone receptor-positive advanced breast cancer (that had progressed or recurred during treatment with an aromatase inhibitor) to exemestane with or without the mTOR inhibitor everolimus. Here are the results after half of patients had been followed for at least 18 months: The median progression free survival was significantly longer with everolimus plus exemestane at 11 versus 4.1 months.

Side effects more common in the everolimus group included infections, rash, lung inflammation, elevated blood sugar and stomatitis (inflammation of the mouth and lips). Elderly patients treated with an everolimus-containing regimen had similar incidences of these adverse events, but the younger patients had more on-treatment deaths.

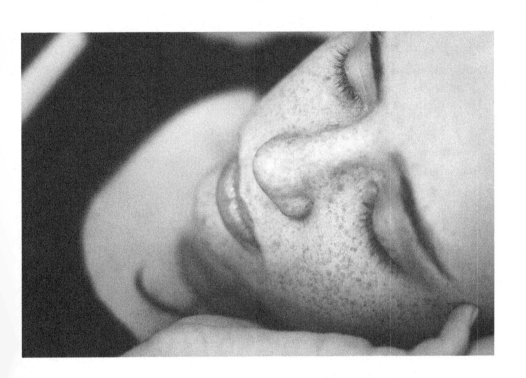

Metastases

Distant spread of cancer

Visceral disease (for example, in the lungs or liver)

Chemotherapy is often perceived as being associated with a higher response rate than anti-estrogen (endocrine) approaches. Still, endocrine therapy is sometimes offered to select patients with disease in solid organs such as the liver or lungs, provided the patient is not in a crisis.

Endocrine therapy (if you cancer is hormone receptor positive*)

In crisis

If you are in a crisis (for example, you have replacement of your bone marrow with cancer, carcinomatous meningitis (a serious in which cancer cells spread from the breast to the meninges - thin layers of tissue that cover and protect the brain and spinal cord), a significant volume of cancer in your liver, or lymphangitic lung metastases**), chemotherapy is generally recommended in order to try to achieve rapid symptom relief.

Not in crisis

The National Comprehensive Cancer Network observes that because systemic treatment of metastatic breast cancer can improve survival and enhance quality of life (but is not curative), use of anti-estrogen (endocrine) therapy is *preferred*, when reasonable. Still, if you have symptoms from spread to organs such as the lung or liver, chemotherapy should be strongly considered.

---

* Estrogen receptor positive and/or progesterone receptor positive (ER+ and/or PR+)
** A condition in which cancer cells spread from the original (primary) tumor and invade lymph vessels (thin tubes that carry lymph and white blood cells through the body's lymph system). The invaded lymph vessels then fill up with cancer cells and become blocked.

Metastases: Distant spread of cancer

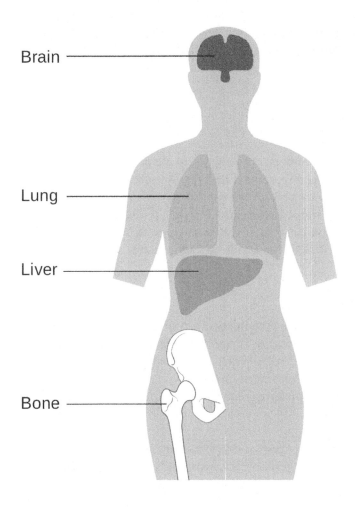

Brain

Lung

Liver

Bone

Predicting response

Metastases: Associated survival

Data from Helsinki (Finland) are illustrative, with researchers finding a **median breast cancer-specific survival time after recurrence of 2.7 years** for breast cancer in general (not specific to inflammatory breast cancer). This means that fully half of patients will live beyond that number. Survival odds appeared better for those who had Stage I disease initially, compared to those with more advanced stages.

Predicting response

Two of the most important predictors of response to treatment include receptor status (estrogen receptor (ER), progesterone receptor (PR), and HER2). Having a breast cancer that is ER-positive is associated with a response to anti-estrogen (endocrine) treatment, while HER2 overexpression is linked to a potential response to anti-HER2 strategies such as trastazumab (Herceptin), pertuzumab (Perjeta), lapatinib, and ado-trastuzumab emtansine (Kadcyla).

Chemotherapy

You may have a lower probability of a response to chemotherapy if you have had progression after prior chemotherapy for metastatic breast cancer. Other predictors of a lower response chance include: 1) a greater number of metastatic sites; 2) involvement of so-called visceral structures (for example, the liver or lung); 3) you have great challenges in your day-to-day life (poor performance status).

Markers suggesting a higher rate of cancer cell division (high proliferation) portend a favorable response to chemotherapy. These features include a high S-phase fraction and/or a high Ki-67 proliferation index.

Invasive

Management: "Bone hardening" drugs

Bisphosphonates and RANK-ligand inhibitors

Bone-modifying agents (including bisphosphonates and the so-called RANK-ligand inhibitor denosumab) have a clear role in the management of patients with breast cancer spread to the bones, and are even used to to reduce the risk for bone fractures among high-risk populations without cancer. What is not entirely clear is the role of these drugs as a component of treatment for early stage breast cancer. A recent analysis of randomized trials suggests a role for these agents in women with breast cancer who have gone through menopause. Let's look at the takeaway lessons from this meta-analysis that included data from 18,766 women in 26 clinical trials:

> • In consultation between the patient and oncologist, bisphosphonates should be considered for women after menopause with breast cancer who are considered candidates for systemic therapy. Disease charac teristics and risk factors for breakdown of the jaw bone (osteonecrosis) and kidney function impairment should be considered.

> • Zoledronic acid (every 6 months for 3 to 5 years) and clodronate (daily) are the recommended bisphophonates.

> • A dental assessment is recommended prior to starting bisphophosphonate therapies.

Metastases

Distant spread of cancer

Brain metastases

The brain is increasingly reported as the first site of relapse among women with HER-2 positive breast cancer treated with trastazumab (Herceptin).

Management: Favorable prognosis

If you have a "favorable" prognosis (that is, you have a Karnofsky Performance Status of 70 or higher*; have a controlled primary cancer, controlled (or absent) metastases outside of the brain, and are under 65 year old), aggressive management is typically offered.

For example, if you have only a single site of spread in the brain, you may have the metastasis removed surgically, followed by radiation therapy (often highly focused, high-dose rather than whole brain) versus highly focused radiation therapy (radiosurgery) alone. Let's look in more detail at the management for those with a limited number (for example, 1 to 3) of metastases in the brain.

Limited volume brain metastases

For those who are in the "favorable" prognosis group, and who have a limited number/volume of brain metastases, here are some of your options:

- **Surgery**

  If you have a single, large metastases in an area of the brain that is accesible to a neurosurgeon, surgery may offer the best chance for rapid symptom relief and control of the cancer in that particular area. You may also be offered surgery if you have more than one metastasis in the brain, but there is one that is dominant and causing you distressing symptoms. Finally, if cancer in the brain is blocking the fluid drainage system in and around the brain, a tube might be placed to bypass the blockage. We call this tube a shunt.

- **Stereotactic radiosurgery (SRS)**

Stereotactic radiosurgery (high doses of highly focused radiation therapy, given in as few as 1 to 3 treatments) can be a a very effective alternative to surgery. You may be a candidate for this innovative form of radiation therapy if you metastasis is relatively small (say, smaller than 3 cm) and in a location that is suboptimal for surgery, or if you are not a candidate for surgery of the brain. SRS may still be an option even if you have more than 3 tumors in the brain.

- **Whole brain radiation therapy (WBRT)**

Historically, whole brain radiation therapy was the mainstay of treatment for metastases to the brain. It continues to play multiple roles in the modern era; for example. it may be used when surgery or stereotactic radiosurgery (SRS) are not feasible (say, too many metastases in the brain).

- **Systemic Therapy**

Systemic therapy (for example, chemotherapy or trastazumab (Herceptin)) is not typically used as primary therapy for brain metastases. If the spread to the brain is small in volume, and the patient has no symptoms, radiation therapy may sometimes be delayed, in favor of continuing drugs such as Herceptin.

Metastases

Distant spread of cancer

Brain metastases: In more detail

Surgery with or without whole brain radiation therapy

For solitary brain metastases, upfront resection remains the standard of care. A randomized trial for 95 patients with a single brain metastasis compared a complete resection alone with surgery followed by radiation therapy to the whole brain. The addition of whole brain radiation therapy dropped the in-brain recurrence rate from 70 percent to 18 percent, and lowered the chances of a neurologic death from 44 percent to 14 percent.

The addition (to surgery) of radiation therapy did *not* improve survival length, however. If you have multiple metastases to the brain, the role of surgery may be limited to obtaining biopsy samples or relieving mass effect when tumors are large. Resection may be offered to highly selected patients with up to three metastases in the brain.

Stereotactic radiosurgery (SRS) with or without whole brain radiation therapy

This innovative form of radiation therapy offers a minimally invasive alternative to surgery for selected individuals with a limited volume of metastases in the brain. We have growing evidence to suggest that the key determinant in whether you are a candidate for SRS is the volume (rather than the number) of metastases in the brain. SRS is often delivered in one to three sessions.

The Choosing Wisely campaign offers that we should *not* routinely add *whole brain* radiation therapy after stereotactic radiosurgery for limited brain metastases. The addition of whole brain radiation therapy to stereotactic radiosurgery is associated with diminished cognitive function and worse patient-reported fatigue and quality of life.

A Japanese randomized study of patients with 1 to 4 brain metastases (smaller than 3 cm) showed that the addition of whole brain radiation therapy to SRS did *not* improve survival. However, the 1-year in-brain recurrence rate was lower (47%) with SRS plus whole brain radiation therapy, compared to SRS alone (76%). A meta-analysis (study of a collection of studies) found **no overall survival improvement with the addition of whole brain radiation therapy to stereotactic radiosurgery.**

Recurrence in brain after whole brain radiation therapy

Local control rates greater than 70% have been reported for individuals who receive stereotactic radiosurgery in the setting of recurrence following whole brain radiation therapy. Stereotactic radiosurgery (SRS) may be offered if you are otherwise doing reasonably well (good performance status), and have relatively stable cancer elsewhere.

Whole brain radiation therapy

Historically whole brain radiation represented the gold standard treatment for brain metastases. We still use it, particularly when surgery or stereotactic radiosurgery is not prudent. While we don't have randomized trials, case series point to up to 70% of patients deriving symptom relief from radiation therapy. Typically, a radiation therapy course for brain metastases is 2 to 3 weeks, Monday through Friday. This corresponds to 30 Gy ("gray") in 10 treatments or 37.5 Gy in 15 treatments. You will be in the radiation therapy department less than half an hour typically, and the treatment itself takes only minutes.

Systemic therapy

Chemotherapy is *not* typically offered as primary management of brain metastases, unless other reasonable options have been exhausted. Highly selected patients without symptoms may have systemic therapy, delaying radiotherapy.

Surveillance

After whole brain radiation therapy or stereotactic radiosurgery patients should have a **repeat MRI scan every 3 months for a year.** If recurrence in the brain occurs and you have systemic (body) progression with limited systemic treatment options, you may choose palliative/best supportive care or reirradiation. For those with stable systemic (body) disease, options may include surgery, reirradiation, or chemotherapy.

Metastases

Distant spread of cancer

Leptomeningeal metastases

This refers to multifocal spread of cancer to the membranes (meninges) surrounding the brain and spinal cord. We sometimes refer to it as leptomeningeal carcinomatosis or carcinomatous meningitis when the cancer has spread from a solid tumor such as is the case for breast cancer. The cancer cells gain access to the leptomeninges through the bloodstream, lymph system, or by direct extension. Once they enter the cerebrospinal fluid, they can disseminate throughout the central nervous system. Many patients develop problems with the nerves that supply the face and head (cranial nerves), headaches, mental changes, or motor weakness. Unfortunately, the median survival is measured in months.

Management

Treatment intervention is aimed at improving or stabilizing neurologic function, and to prolong survival. There is no standard approach, but radiation therapy may be offered for symptom relief, to shrink the tumor burden (for the select patient who will get chemotherapy), or to allow the cerebrospinal fluid to flow more normally. Surgery is limited primarily to placement of a catheter into the brain ventricles (reservoirs of spinal fluid in the central brain) for drug administration.

Chemotherapy may be offered, as it can reach the central nervous system. Alternatively, the direct delivery of drugs may be offered either by a catheter placed in the spine region (intrathecal therapy), or through a device your neurosurgeon can implant directly into your brain's ventricles (pools of spinal fluid in the central brain). Breast cancer may then respond to drugs such as methotrexate or trastazumab (Herceptin). At Memorial Sloan Kettering Cancer Center (USA), the half of patients lived beyond 3.5 months, with 20% surviving more than a year.

Brain metatases: Outcomes

(in general; *not specific to inflammatory breast cancer*)

	Median survival
ER negative, HER2 negative	27 months
HER2 positive	52 months
ER positive, HER2 negative, Ki-67 high	76 months
ER positive, HER2 negative, Ki-67 low	79 months

Brain metastases: Neuroprotective strategies

Unfortunately, whole brain radiation therapy can result in a decline in your brain function (neurocognitive changes). A a result, researchers are working hard to find ways of reducing risk. Here are some examples of these strategies:

Memantine (Namenda)

Memantine is a drug that is sometimes offered for Alzheimer's disease. It can delay the time to cognitive decline. More recently, we have begun to use it for patients receiving whole brain radiation therapy.

In a randomized trial compared memantine (beginning 3 days prior to radiation therapy, and continuing for 24 weeks) or a placebo. The time to cognitive decline appeared longer for the group on memantine. Recognizing the effectiveness of the drug, and its relatively favorable side effect profile, you may wish to consider this drug if you are to receive whole brain radiation therapy.

Hippocampal-sparing radiation therapy

Using a highly advanced form of radiation therapy known as intensity modulated radiation therapy (IMRT), one can attempt to avoid radiation injury to the hippocampus. This structure plays an important role in the formation of new memories about experienced events (episodic or autobiographical memory). This approach requires a great deal of treatment planning, including robust physics team support. As it is relatively new, most patients do not have this approach.

Breast cancer may spread to brain by masquerading as nerve cells

City of Hope scientists wanted to explore how breast cancer cells cross the blood-brain barrier – a separation of the blood circulating in the body from fluid in the brain – without being destroyed by the immune system. If, by chance, a malignant breast cancer cell swimming in the bloodstream crossed into the brain, how would it survive in a completely new, foreign habitat?

Taking samples from brain tumors resulting from breast cancer, researchers found that the breast cancer cells were exploiting the brain's most abundant chemical as a fuel source. This chemical (GABA) is a neurotransmitter used for communication between neurons.

When compared to cells from non-metastatic breast cancer, the metastasized cells expressed a receptor for GABA, as well as for a protein that draws the transmitter into cells. This allowed the cancer cells to essentially masquerade as neurons."Breast cancer cells can be cellular chameleons (or masquerade as neurons) and spread to the brain," lead researcher Dr. Jandial offered.
Jandial says that further study is required to better understand the mechanisms that allow the cancer cells to achieve this disguise. He hopes that ultimately, unmasking these disguised invaders will result in new therapies.

In-brain recurrence (after initial treatment of brain metastases)
If you have stable disease outside of the brain (and are in relatively good condition overall), potential options for re-treatment of brain metastases may include surgery and stereotactic radiosurgery.

Surgery: Results
Re-operation for recurrent brain metastases can sometimes help:

Symptom relief	75%
Median survival	1 year

Radiosurgery for recurrence in brain
A series of 111 patients who had previously received whole brain radiation therapy and were treated with radiosurgery after recurrence of their brain metastases. Of these, 25 percent recurred again after radiosurgery. The median survival after salvage radiosurgery was 10 months.

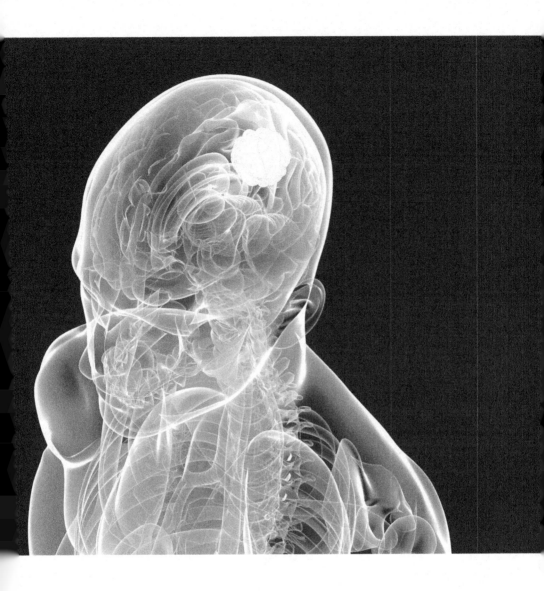

CAR-T cells

Researchers at City of Hope (USA) have opened a first-in-human clinical trial to assess the use of chimeric antigen receptor T-cell (CAR-T) therapy for patients with HER2-positive breast cancer that has spread to the brain. Here, immune system cells are removed from the body, genetically re-engineered to be more effective, and injected back in.

Metastases

Oligometastases

Very limited distant spread

Are we broadening the path to cure? Many patients who are diagnosed with cancer either present with or will develop distant metastatic cancer. in general, metastatic disease is considered incurable, so there are two ways in which we may increase cancer cure rates: 1) improve our diagnosis and management of cancer before it can spread; and 2) discover means to cure metastatic breast cancer.

Emerging data indicate that patients with metastasis to a **limited number of sites (termed oligometastatic disease)** may have improved outcomes with the use of locally ablative therapy (LAT). Historically, when the only management tool for cancer was surgery, the groundbreaking surgeon William Halstead offered a theory of cancer progression, first published in the early 1900s. According to his paradigm, cancer spreads in an orderly fashion initially through the lymphatic system. Therefore, once beyond the localized lymphatic drainage bed, cancer was a systemic disease for which there was no cure. For the most part, this perspective continues to hold true, with some exceptions including germ cell tumors and lymphomas.

Clinical experience, however, has shown that not all patients with metastases have widely disseminated disease. Hellman and Weichselbaum more recently proposed that cancer metastases fall on a continuum. Although some cancers feature either localized or disseminated characteristics, most fall between these extremes. Some tumors may metastasize to a limited number of sites, a condition we call oligometastatic cancer. In general, most studies of oligometastatic cancer have included patients with one to five distinct metastases. With a limited number of metastases, it becomes theoretically possible to treat all detectable tumors with curative intent using locally ablative therapy (LAT). With increasingly more advanced imaging techniques, we should improve our ability to find metastatic disease when it is early and limited, giving more hope to many with metastases.

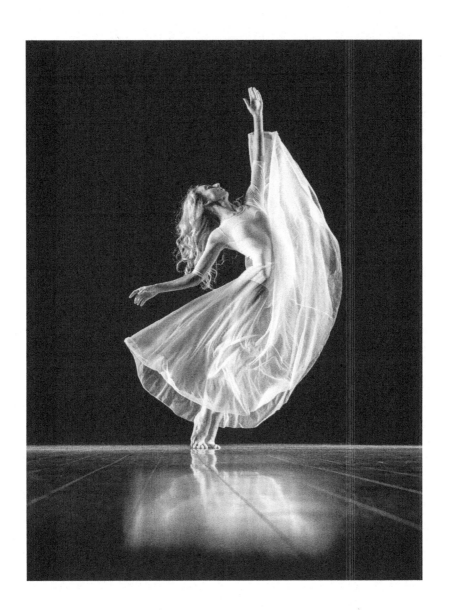

Metastases

Distant spread of cancer

The Association of Community Cancer Centers (acc-cancer.org/Metastatic-BreastCancer) offers effective principles in metastatic cancer patient support. Let's take a look:

• Empower

Given the terminal nature of metastatic breast cancer, you may feel that the disease has stripped you of control. Life goals may start to feel less achievable, and because life expectancies are highly variable from person to person, you may not feel comfortable navigating conversations with family, friends, and co-workers. In order to try to empower you, oncology providers should communicate information to you in a way that does not rely on overly complex language. As a clinician, I try to strike a balance between honesty and hope - allowing you to understand the reality and then decide how to move forward.

• Include

Often, individuals with metastatic breast cancer feel excluded from the dominant breast cancer narrative. There seems to be a significant lack of understanding of the unique issues for those in this population. Unfortunately, many in the public rely on their understanding of early breast cancer to navigate conversations with patients who have metastatic breast cancer. In addition, some patients perceive the incurable nature of the disease as an immediate death sentence. As caregivers, we should aim to communicate clearly, yet also offer a source of hope.

• Support

Social support can be a key source of psychological and even physical relief. The dominant narrative of early detection and survivorship may lead you to feel that you are going through this process alone. How many of the general population really understand what you are going through when you have metastatic breast cancer? Social support can come in a variety of forms, including retreats,

208

mentorship programs, in-person support groups, phone support groups, and online support groups. Optimally, given challenges in creating social spaces that include both those with metastatic disease and those without it, we need to do a better job of making appropriate spaces for those with metastases to share their experiences and needs.

• Help

The emotional stress of living with metastatic breast cancer produces additional difficulty for patients when they are faced with challenges that they are not informationally or emotionally equipped to handle. Logistical support needs may be in areas such as clinical trials and finances, and stress reduction. By getting help with logistics, you may be better able to focus on important facets of life, including family, extra-curricular activities, and work.

• Connect

Your community may have additional resources, beyond those of your medical center. Ask your care providers about such resources.

In our Seattle community, we are blessed to have extraordinary resources through our Hospice and palliative care programs. Please ask you valued care provider about such resources in your community.

13

AFTER
SURVIVORSHIP

Survivorship

A survivor is defined by me as any person with cancer, starting from the moment of diagnosis. There are 14 million breast cancer survivors in the USA alone, and as many as 29 million worldwide.

Follow-up

I use the National Comprehensive Cancer Network (NCCN) Guidelines, updated regularly by experts from a group of leading cancer managing institutions. There is a patient version too, available online at www.nccn.org. For **invasive** breast cancer in general*, the pathway is as follows:

- History and physical exam 1 to 4 times per year as clinically appropriate for 5 years, then annually

- Periodic screening for changes in family history and referral to genetic counseling as indicated

- Educate, monitor, and refer for lymphedema management

- Mammograms every 12 months [if breast(s) preserved]

- In the absence of clinical signs and symptoms suggestive of recurrent cancer, there is no indication for imaging studies for metastases (distant spread of cancer) screening

- For women on tamoxifen, annual gynecologic assessment (if uterus present)

- For women on an aromatase inhibitor (or who enter menopause because of treatment), there should be monitoring of bone health with a bone mineral density (DEXA) test at baseline, and then periodically

- Encouragement of adherence to endocrine therapy (such as tamoxifen, or aromatase inhibitor pills)

---

* Not specific to inflammatory breast cancer. Also, we do not have a lot of data to inform optimal follow-up for males with breast cancer, and typically apply the aforementioned guidelines.

Cancer surveillance

History and physical examination remain the principle means for detecting a breast cancer recurrence. For patients who have had breast-conserving management, breast imaging is indicated:

- Mammograms

While data is limited, surveillance mammograms for residual breast tissue after breast conserving treatment, or for the contralateral breast (after a mastectomy for one side) appears to lower breast cancer mortality. There is indirect evidence from retrospective series that supports a benefit for mammograms of the opposite (contralateral) breast. Some advocate no imaging for those with a life expectancy of under 5 to 10 years.

- Breast MRI

Breast magnetic resonance imaging is not routinely recommended for breast cancer survivors. Still, breast MRI can be of value for patients suspected of having a breast cancer recurrence, or when the mammogram is inconclusive.

- Ultrasound

Routine use of ultrasound is not recommended.

- Reconstructed breasts

For those who have had a breast removal or mastectomy, surveillance is primarily via physical examination. Routine mammograms are not done for those with prostetic implants. While mammograms are technically possible after a TRAM flap reconstruction, there is no consensus on whether to do them or not, as we do not have much evidence to guide us. Still, physical examination can be invaluable in detecting a local recurrence.

Bone density

Women with a history of breast cancer can have a higher risk of developing bone loss, including osteoporosis, as a result of cancer treatment. In this context, the American Society of Clinical Oncology (ASCO) recommends a baseline screening evaluation (typically with a dual energy X-ray absorptiometry, or DEXA scan) for those over 65 years of age, for those 60 to 64 who have a family history of osteoporosis, those with a body weight under 154 pounds (70 kg), a history of a non-traumatic fracture, or other risk factors (such as smoking, alcohol use, or a sedentary lifestyle).

Blood work and imaging

For breast cancer survivors without symptoms, routine laboratory surveillance (or imaging) is *not* recommended. Here, we have high-level evidence: A 2005 meta-analysis two randomized trials that compared routine follow-up (physical exam and mammograms) versus intensive surveillance (including imaging and blood tests) showed no differences between the groups in overall or disease-free survival odds.

Routine tumor marker testing

The 2012 American Society of Clinical Oncology (ASCO) Guidelines offer the following: The use of CA 15-3 or CA 27.29 is *not* recommended for routine surveillance of patients following primary management for breast cancer. CEA is also not recommended.

Circulating tumor cells (CTCs)

The current evidence does *not* support the use or circulating tumor cells (CTCs) to evaluate for recurrence after treatment for primary breast cancer. While the presence of CTCs has indeed been linked with poorer prognosis, we have only limited data.

Lifestyle

My patients frequently ask what they can do to optimize their prognosis from breast cancer. Lifestyle modification can be an effective and empowering way to enhance physical and psychological well-being, and may improve your disease free- and overall survival opportunities.

Soy: Okay to eat

I am unaware of evidence to suggest that dietary soy (which contains phytoestrogens) affects breast cancer recurrence rates.

Alcohol: Increases risk

We do not have many studies linking alcohol consumption with of recurrence. Still, the largest study showed that those who drank the equivalent of at least 3 to 4 standard drinks (more than 6 grams) of alcohol per week had a 1.35-fold higher risk of recurrence and and 1.5-fold increase in breast cancer death risk, compared to those who consumed less than 0.5 grams daily. The risk among overweight and postmenopausal women appeared highest, in this Life After Cancer Epidemiology (LACE) study.

Complementary

A comprehensive overview of this topic is beyond the scope of this book. The Society for Integrative Oncology (SIO) produced an evidence-based guideline on integrative therapies for the management of symptoms such as anxiety and stress, mood disorders, fatigue, chemotherapy-induced nausea and vomiting, lymphedema, chemotherapy-induced neuropathy, pain, and sleep disturbance.

The American Society of Clinical Oncology (ASCO) expert panel endorsed this guideline. Key recommendations include: Music therapy, meditation, stress management and yoga for anxiety and stress reduction. Meditation, relaxation, yoga, massage, and music therapy are recommended for depression/mood disorders. Meditation and yoga are recommended to improve quality of life. Acupressure and acupuncture are recommended for reducing chemotherapy-induced nausea and vomiting. No strong evidence supports the use of ingested dietary supplements to manage breast cancer treatment-related side effects.

Physical activity, body weight, and diet

Observational studies show an association between survival and physical activity, with most of the data involving patients with breast, colon, or prostate cancer.

A meta-analysis of 16 prospective observational trials showed a near halving (48 percent reduction) in overall mortality and a 28 percent drop in breast cancer mortality in the most versus least active breast cancer survivors. Breast cancer survivors who increased their activity after diagnosis (relative to pre-diagnosis levels) dropped their mortality by more than a third (39 percent relative risk reduction).

Exercise can also help improve aerobic fitness, quality of life, strength, anxiety and depression, fatigue, body image, and body size and composition. It is not clear what the best exercise type is, but many of my patients aim for moderate activity such as a brisk walk for 30 minutes, five days per week.

Weight loss

Two large trials have looked at the benefits of weight loss among women with breast cancer. The Lifestyle Intervention Study for Adjuvant Treatment of Early Breast Cancer (LISA) randomly assigned 338 post-menopausal women with hormone receptor-positive breast cancer to a two-year telephone-based weight loss intervention or to usual care. The telephone group lost 5.4 percent weight by one year, and 3.7 percent at two years. The control group lost less (0.7 and 0.4 percent, respectively). In addition, those in the intervention group significantly improved their physical functioning. The Exercise and Nutrition to Enhance Recovery and Good Health for You (ENERGY) trial confirmed these results. We look forward to determining whether such weight loss improves breast cancer outcomes, as there are a number of trials looking at that.

Hot flashes

We generally avoid estrogen and progesterone for those with a history of breast cancer. Some patients with severe symptoms may benefit from non-hormonal drugs suh as gabapentin in the evening or so-called serotonin reuptake inhibitors (SSRIs)/serotonin norepinephrine reuptake inhibitors (SNRIs). Some have concerns about interactions with tamoxifen, however. In this context, many avoid paroxetine or fluoxetine, but may use other drugs such as citalopram or venlafaxine.

Acupuncture has shown promising results in some clinical trials, with one study showing it works better than the drug gabapentin. A Wake Forest Baptist Medical Center (USA) study found that acupuncture reduced hot flashes and night sweats by over a third, with this benefit lasting for at least six months.

Depression and libido

Depression is a common result of breast cancer management, and can in turn affect sexuality. If you are depressed, please let your care team know. Many patients turn to therapists or group support. Antidepressant medications are sometimes offered, but this needs to be done in consultation with your medical oncologist; some medicines may affect drugs such as tamoxifen. For example, paroxetin (Paxil), buproprion (Wellbutrin), Prozac, duloxetine (Cymbalta) and Zoloft may challenge your body's ability to convert tamoxifen into its active form, potentially reducing the full benefits of tamoxifen.

If loss of libido is an issue for you, you may be a candidate for testosterone (the primary hormone in men). However, if your testosterone levels are within normal limits, more testosterone will not likely provide a benefit to you. Finally, treatment-induced nausea can understandably take away your interest in sex.

Vaginal dryness

Menopause, whether natural or treatment-caused, may result in thinning and shortening of your vaginal walls. There can be associated dryness, or lack of vaginal lubrication which can lead to pain associated with sex. Some find relief with topical lidocaine. The American Society of Clinical Oncology (ASCO) recommends the use of non-hormonal treatments, including water- or silicone-based lubricants or moisturizers as first line treatment for vaginal dryness and pain associated with sex. Vaginal moisturizers include products containing gelatins, gums, polycarbophil, or hyaluronic acid.

Lymphedema (arm swelling)

Lymphedema (edema) is defined as the collection of protein-rich fluid in spaces within a tissue, due to disruption of the flow of lymph fluid. Lymphedema is an overflow problem: The lymph load exceeds the transport capacity of the lymphatic system. Unfortunately, this swelling (for example of the arm) can be associated with surgery or radiation therapy. It can manifest as slowly progressive swelling of the arm, and can also include the breast or upper chest wall.

In a systematic review of 72 studies, the overall incidence of arm edema among survivors of breast cancer was 17 percent. Risk factors for breast cancer associated lymphedema (arm swelling) include the following:

Axillary node dissection
The surgical removal of nodes is the primary cause of breast and arm swelling, with the incidence increasing with the number of axillary nodes removed or disrupted. The risk is around 20 percent for those who have an axillary node dissection (removal of several nodes from a geographic zone), compared to 5.6 percent for thos having a sentinel node biopsy.

Radiation therapy (RT)
Lympedema risk appears is much higher if you have had axillary dissection *and* radiation therapy, as compared with axillary dissection alone. In one systematic review, the risk of edema was 41 percent with both, compared to 17 percent with surgery alone. Radiation therapy field design affects risk, too: More comprehensive radiotherapy volumes covering more of the axilla, nodes around the collarbone, and nodes next to the breast bone can further increase risk, compared to more limited RT.

Other
Excessive body weight (body mass index) can increase edema risk, as can infections after surgery, blood or fluid collections after surgery, and possibly medications such as chemotherapy. Weight gain can put you at additional risk, as it may impair lymphatic function.

The breast cancer management type may affect the timing of the development of lymphedema. It appears that early-onset edema (less than one year after surgery) may be more associated with surgery, while late-onset lymphedema seems more associated with radiation therapy to regional lymph nodes.

Lymphedema risk reduction

Primary prevention

A sentinel node sampling (rather than a more thorough axillary node dissection) is a primary means of reducing risk, but is *not* currently used for inflammatory breast cancer. Sophisticated radiotherapy techniques may lower risk, too, as may surgical techniques such as reverse mapping or lymphatic bypass.

Secondary prevention

Here, the goal is to control arm swelling. We often monitor arm circumference. I ask patients to maintain excellent skin and nail care, as infection can lead to skin inflammation (cellulitis). A good skin moisturizer may help, as can protection of your hands with gloves when you are participating in activities that may lead to skin injury. If you have any signs of infection, report them.

Many patients benefit from elevation of the arm, particularly in the early stages of edema. Properly fitted compression sleeves may help. In addition, try to avoid procedures (for examples, blood draws or vaccinations) that puncture the skin of the arm. Blood pressure measurements are best done using the opposite arm. Finally, try to maintain a good body weight, preferably with a body mass index of 20 to 25.

Travel

Given the lower atmospheric pressure at altitude, the risk from air travel precipitating or worsening edema is present, but is fortunately low. Some patients use compression sleeves during air travel, but I do not think there is consensus on whether this is required, particularly with flights under about 4.5 hours.

Exercises

We typically offer our patients (who have had any surgery of nodes) range of motion exercises for the affected arm. After you have healed following surgery, exercise (including weight training) appears to be safe and even beneficial. Early physiotherapy such as manual lymphatic drainage can provide benefit.

Surgery

Surgery may aid highly select patients with lymphedema, and may help with pain. It appears to work best for those with early-stage lymphedema.

Left untreated the degree of lymphedema typically increases over time. Conservative management may include:

Compression therapy

Often combined with physiotherapy, compression therapy may be offered for early lymphedema. Limb compression and the use of fitted compression garments may play roles, some benefit from use of an appropriately fitted compression hand piece (such as a glove).

Manual lymphatic drainage

MLD may provide additional benefits (although this is controversial), when added to compression therapy. This massage-like approach is done by a specially trained physical therapist. A systematic review of six trials concluded that the approach is safe, and may offer additional benefit to compression bandaging for swelling reduction. Those with mild-to-moderate lymphedema appear to be the ones who benefit from adding manual lymphatic drainage to an intensive course of compression bandaging.

Intermittent pneumatic compression

This is another method of compression therapy. It is most typically offered to those with severe lymphedema. Unfortunately, we do not have high level evidence regarding its effectiveness, but some have concerns about pressures greater than 60 mmHg.

Complete decongestive therapy

This technique may be recommended if you have moderate-to-severe lymphedema. A small trial randomized patients to CDT (including lymph drainage, multilayer compression bandaging, elevation, remedial exercise, and skin care) versus standard physiotherapy (elevation, bandages, head/neck/shoulder exercises, and skin care) found a greater improvement in lymphedema with the more intense approach. However, a second similar study found no such benefit.

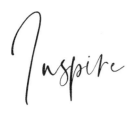

Inspire

My story

I'm Nancy, and this is my story. For me, it began with a common garden spider bite. Or so I thought. Days later I noticed the bites on my side were gone, but the one on my breast was not. Still, no real concern, even though it itched like crazy. A week or so later, again in the shower, my attention heightened as I noticed that the skin around the bump was thick and dimpled like an orange peel. Now that got my attention. I was concerned that it may have been a poison spider and the skin was dying. I called my ob/gyn to have it checked and I was scheduled to see her the following week. And so I went down the rabbit hole.

After a physical exam, I immediately got mammograms and a breast ultrasound, even though I had just had a "normal" mammo a couple of months earlier. During the ultrasound the imaging doctor said there was a blockage in the lymph system, but as he could not determine the cause, more tests would be needed. As I left his office to walk across the hall to my ob/gyn, his nurse took my hand and in a low, serious voice said "good luck to you, honey." The hairs on the back of my neck stood on end. My doctor's nurse told me that she had made me an appointment with a surgeon. The next afternoon I met with a lovely young surgeon who took a biopsy of the lymphatic blockage and the thickened skin.

Surreal

I kept thinking "What, there must be some mistake!" The doctor told me the time frame for my treatment, with the first of six rounds of chemo to begin a week later, followed by a modified radical mastectomy, provided the oncologist was pleased with the effectiveness of the chemo. Then, a month recovery from surgery, six more rounds of a different type of chemo again at three week intervals to be followed by 26 to 30 radiation treatments. "Do you have any questions?" Questions? I didn't even know what half of what she was saying meant, I had never heard of this disease, my head was spinning and I was sure I was going to faint! My husband scooped me up and we drove home in a deafening silence. **He gave me comfort.**

The next day, we met my oncologist. She was serious and matter of fact about the next eleven months of my life, letting me know that this was not going to be an easy process and would be fraught with side effects, including discomfort and pain. She advised me not to read about inflammatory breast cancer on the internet or in hard copy, explaining that all I would find was the consensus that I was probably going to die. She did not believe that was the most likely outcome for me, given recent changes in management. **She gave me hope.**

After days of testing, my husband and I arrived at the hospital to prep for the outpatient surgery for my port. As I was sat on the side of the bed waiting for the nurse to tell me what to do, I thought about my last few weeks, going from being a happy housewife working in the garden to a cancer patient shivering and scared. My life and those of my family had flipped dramatically. When the nurse came in to begin my IV I was washed over by a wave of terror. This was real, it wasn't a mistake! As I silently wept, the nurse took my hand and squeezed. **She gave me strength.**

So the routine began. Chemotherapy infusions that took four to five hours, then home to rest. About five hours after chemo I was overwhelmed with nausea. It would come in waves, so I spent the majority of my time on the couch or in the bathroom. The nausea medication was promptly thrown up, with suppositories giving only minimal relief. The second week was better, but I felt as though I was in a boat in the middle of a perfect storm. That week, at least I could eat a little, but something in the chemo made my mouth sore and everything I tried to eat tasted metallic, but most of what I could force down stayed down. The third week was pretty good, not much nausea, and a tiny flicker of energy, but I knew that more chemo was only a few days away!

I was overwhelmed and sure I had ruined the lives of my family members. I could not care for my three year old grandson, my daughter had to hurriedly find day care, my husband was stressed and scared, and it was all my fault. I wasn't sure I was going to be able to do it. Seventeen days into my first round of chemo and in the middle of the night, the house was cold and dark and silent. My husband was sleeping, I had taken a pillow and blanket into the bathroom so I didn't disturb him, since I was in there most of the time anyway. As I laid my head on the side of the tub to try to rest after puking and crying, it dawned on me, I had to take control of this! I began to think of ways I could do that, I couldn't do anything about the drugs and side effects, so why not think of them in a different way. I decided to see vomiting as throwing up cancer cells, my hair was falling out so that meant the chemo was working.

Inspire

On the morning after my second round of chemo, I awakened with a severely swollen arm. It was so swollen that the skin was tight, and it looked like a giant sausage. I drove myself to the cancer center, which was only three minutes from my house. When I walked in you would have thought I had an axe in my head, everyone began to run around me, talking rapidly, putting me in a wheelchair and rushing me to the intensive care unit. I had developed a blood clot at the end of the tube of the Port-a-Cath. I had a day getting treatments to reduce the clot, spent the night in the hospital with my arm wrapped in ice, and the next morning had the old port taken out and a new one put in a larger artery. After this short break the mundane process resumed.

The chemo routine went on for about three months, and each time before my next round the oncologist would ask if I wanted her to reduce the dosage. I was pretty sure I could survive treatment, and I was very sure I could not survive the disease absent effective management, so I never backed it down. My energy was gone because my body was busy killing cancer. Surprisingly, that decision changed a lot for me emotionally. **I gave myself perseverance.**

I met with the surgeon about the mastectomy, and I wanted her to cut off both of my breasts. That seemed logical and easier than dealing with prostheses each time I would be with people. She disagreed, offering that she would take lymph nodes from the cancer side, and really didn't want to disturb the ones on the other side. I fought for my plan, but she convinced me it was wiser to get a breast reduction instead. So I met with a plastic surgeon for that procedure. I explained to him that I wanted to be as small as I could, flat even. He insisted that he would make my breast pretty, in case I wanted reconstruction on the other side in the future. I did not, as my docs had told me to avoid covering the chest wall, given recurrence is so likely with inflammatory breast cancer.

The surgeries were performed at the same time and when I awakened, my surgeon was standing next to my bed holding my hand. She turned to me, asking "Doesn't it feel good to know the cancer is gone?". I just closed my eyes and listened. But mostly this chemo made me so tired and achy, it would hurt to just watch my husband walk. Back to the couch I went.

The next three months brought a different type of chemo. This one didn't upset my stomach, but it made my bones ache. For three days before each infusion I had to take a steroid, so my body would tolerate the chemo. The steroid made me feel jittery, like I was about to jump out of my skin, but too tired to move. My eyes jiggled, so reading was out, and watching television marginal.

I did not know what to expect with radiation therapy, but the kindest doctor guided me through the process with grace. These treatments were every weekday for six weeks. They sapped my energy and blistered my skin, but with a calm stomach they were tolerable. On the day of my last radiation therapy, the staff presented a placard and balloons to commemorate my completion of radiotherapy. I was thrilled, and yet frightened. What would I do now? Who would I talk with for my questions? I could not just go back to my previous life, I was not the same person. I asked my doc and she said "Go live your life." I had no idea what that meant. **She gave me possibilities.**

About halfway through my treatment I joined a support group for breast cancer. The ladies were understanding, helpful, and we often ended up in bouts of laughter. These survivors taught me that there was life after all this mayhem, and it could be a darn good one, just not the one I had before. By the time my treatment was over, I was sure that these lovely sisters of breast cancer were the most alive people that I had ever known, and I wanted to be that too. I can honestly say that my life now is better, different yes, but better than it has ever been. **I had hope.**

I appreciate each day, have truly learned how to play, and love more preciously than when I was "normal." I am aware every day how lucky I am that I survived this horrid disease. I have attended too many funerals of lovely women that I have met on this journey to ever forget. I am vigilant of my health, staying fit and helping my immune system function as efficiently as possible. I am sure that I have survived due to the fact that my doctor knew what IBC was from the very beginning and rushed me into treatment. **She gave me life.**

My story began seventeen years ago.

Final thoughts

by Michael Hunter MD

Thank you for allowing me to enter your life with this book. I hope that it has been valuable. Herein, I have tried to be clear in presenting information critical to you. I ask that you provide feedback, in person or via www.newcancer-info.com.

As we close, I ask that you pursue, wherever possible, management strategies that are evidence-based. In this way, you optimize the chances of having the best care, while reducing your chances of potential harm. Now that we have addressed management, what more can you do that may reduce your chances for a return (progression) of the cancer?

- Have a balanced diet
- Optimize of your body: mass index
- Be prudent with alcohol consumption
- Try to be compliant with endocrine therapy, if you are on it.
- Avoid tobacco
- Get some physical activity

I wish you all the best, and feel privileged to communicate with you through this book. You may also find me at www.newcancerinfo.com. **Thank you.**

Oh, one more thing: I often wonder why inflammatory breast cancer seems to be a different (and more aggressive) disease than other breast cancers. Some now believe that there is something present in the microenvironment of some patients that predisposes cancer cells to become more like inflammatory breast cancer rather than "regular" breast cancer. I hope that we may someday target the microenvironment with drugs, or by other means. I am honored to meet individuals who have inflammatory breast cancer, and to be a part of a community dedicated to improving outcomes for those with inflammatory breast cancer.

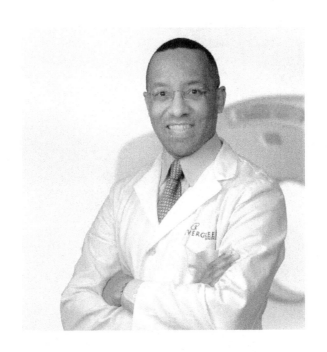

Michael Hunter, MD

Thank you!

EDITING   Maya Hunter (lead editor); Lisa Magnussen RN, OCN, Melissa Pederson RN, OCN; Michelle Trygg, RN, OCN, Lauren Pederson;

IMAGES   pp. 81; 89 Illustrations by Sarah Mahoney Voccola.

p. 67   "Invasive carcinoma of no special type." Wikipedia. Wikipedia.org. n.p., en.wikipedia.org/wiki/Invasive_carcinoma_of_no_special_type. Accessed 2 April 2019.

"Invasive lobular carcinoma." Wikipedia. Wikipedia.org. n.p., en.wikipedia. org/wiki/Invasive_lobular_carcinoma. Accessed 2 April 2019.

CARTOON   p. 127   Immunotherapy cartoon: Courtesy of ACT Genomics (http://www. actgenomics.com/), reprinted with permission.

NOTES

1 basics

1. Breasted JH. The Edwin Smith Surgical Papyrus. Chicago: University of Chicago Press; 1930.
2. http://www.cancer.org/acs/groups/content/@editorial/documents/document/acspc-044552.pdf
3. http://globocan.iarc.fr/Pages/fact_sheets_cancer.aspx, 2014.
4. Stanford, J., Herrinton, L., Schwartz, S., & Weiss, N. (1995). Breast cancer incidence in Asian migrants to the United States and their descendants. Epidemiology, 6, 181–183.
5. Hemminki, K., & Li, X. (2002). Cancer risks in second-generation immigrants to Sweden. Int J Cancer, 99, 229–237.
6. Beiki, O., Hall, P., Ekbom, A., & Moradi, T. (2012). Breast cancer incidence and case fatality among 4.7 million women in relation to social and ethnic background: a population-based cohort study. Breast Cancer Res, 14(1), R5.

Age
7. American Cancer Society, Inc., Surveillance Research, 2017.
8. http://www.targetedonc.com/news/expert-examines-impact-of-age-on-prognosis-molecular-subtype-in-breast-cancer

Race
9. CA: A Cancer Journal for Clinicians. doi: 10.3322/caac.21320. Online at cacancerjournal.com.
10. Keenan T, Moy B, Mroz EA, et al. Comparison of the Genomic Landscape Between Primary Breast Cancer in African American Versus White Women and the Association of Racial Differences With Tumor Recurrence. Presented at the 37th Annual San Antonio Breast Cancer Symposium, San Antonio, TX, December 9-13, 2014, and the 51st Annual Meeting of the American Society of Clinical Oncology, Chicago, IL, May 29-June 2, 2015.
11. American Cancer Society. Cancer Prevention & Early Detection Facts & Figures, 2015-2016.

Genes
12. http://www.cancer.gov/cancertopics/pdq/genetics/breast-and-ovarian/HealthProfessional#sthash.f98eeZ90.dpuf
13. Cancer (2015; doi: 10.1002/cncr.29645)
14. CA Cancer J Clin 2015
15. Walsh T, King MC. Ten genes for inherited breast cancer. Cancer Cell 2007; 11:103-5.
16. Hwang SJ, Lozano G, Amos CI et al. Germline p53 mutations in a cohort with childhood sarcoma: sex differences in cancer risk. Am J Hum Genet 2003; 72(4):975-83.
17. Mouchawar J, Korch C, Byers T et al. Population-based estimate of the contribution of TP53 mutations to subgroups of early-onset breast cancer: Australian Breast Cancer Family Study. Cancer Res 2010; 70(12): 4705-800.
18. Melhem-Bertrandt A, Bojadzieva J, Ready KJ, et al. Early onset HER2-positive breast cancer is associated with germline TP53 mutations. Cancer 2012; 118(4): 908-13.
19. Min-Han T, Mester JL, Ngeow J, et al. Lifetime cancer risks in individuals with germline PTEN mutations. Clin Cancer Res 2012; 18(2): 400-7.
20. Walsh T, King MC. Ten genes for inherited breast cancer. Cancer Cell 2007; 11:103-5.

Radiation exposure
21. Land CE, Tokunaga M, Koyama K et al. Incidence of female breast cancer among atomic bomb survivors. Hiroshima and Nagasaki, 1950-1990. Radiat Res 2003;160: 707-717.
22. Preston DL, Mattsson A, Holmberg E et al. Radiation effects on breast cancer risk for young women treated for Hodgkin lymphoma. J Natl Cancer Inst 2005; 97:1428-37.

Family
23. Collaborative Group on Hormonal Factors in Breast Cancer: Familial breast cancer collaborative reanalysis of individual data from 52 epidemiological studies including 58,209 women with breast cancer and 101,986 women without the disease. Lancet 358: 1389-99, 2001.

Breast density
24. McCormack VA, dos Santos Silva I. Breast density and parenchymal patterns as markers of breast cancer risk: a meta-analysis. Cancer Epidemiol Biomarkers Prev. 2006;15:1159-1569.
25. Katavic N, et al "Association of breast density with breast cancer risk in screening mammography" RSNA Meeting 2015; Abstract BR-5A-01.

Menarche, menopause, height, and obesity
26. Ritte R, et al. Height, age at menarche and risk of hormone receptor-positive and =negative breast cancer as a cohort study. Int J Cancer 2013; 132:2619.
27. Hsieh CC, et al. Age at menarche, age at menopause, height and obesity as risk factors for breast cancer: associations and interactions in an international case-control study. Int J Cancer 1990; 46:796.
28. Collaborative Group on Hormonal Factors in Breast Cancer. Menarche, menopause, and breast cancer risk: individual participant meta-analysis, including 118 964 women with breast cancer from 117 epidemiological studies. Lancet Oncol. 13(11):1141-51, 2012.
29. Colditz GA, et al. Cumulative risk of breast cancer to age 70 years according to risk factor status: data from the Nurses' Health Study. Am J Epidemiol 200; 152:950.

Childbearing; breast-feeding
30. Kelsey JL, et al. Reproductive factors and breast cancer. Epidemiol Rev 1993; 15:36.
31. Rosner B, et al. Reproductive risk factors in a prospective study of breast cancer: the Nurses' Health Study. Am J Epidemiol 1994; 139:814.
32. Annals of Oncology 00: 1–10, 2015 doi:10.1093/annonc/mdv379

Immigrants
33. John EM, Phipps AI, Davis A, Koo J. Migration history, acculturation, and breast cancer risk in Hispanic women. Cancer Epidemiol Biomarkers Prev 2005; 14:2905-13.

Alcohol
34. Alcohol drinking. IARC Working Group, Lyon, 13-20 October 1987. IARC Mongr Eal Carcinog Risks Hum. 1988; 44:1-378.
35. Roswall N, Weiderpass E. Alcohol as a risk factor for cancer: existing evidence in a global perspective. J Prev Med Public Health. 2015; 48:1-9.

Weight gain
36. Newhouser ML et al. JAMA Oncol. 2015;doi:10.1001/jamaoncol.2015.1546.

Risk: Putting it all together (table)
37. Clemons M, et al. N Engl J Med 2001; 344: 276.

Mediterranean diet
38. Estefania T, Salas-Salvado J, Donat-Vargas C, et al. Mediterranean diet and invasive breast cancer risk among women at high cardiovascular risk in the PREDIMED 10.1001.jamainternmed.2015.4838
39. Nutr Rev. 2014 Jan;72(1):1-17. doi: 10.1111/nure.12083. Epub 2013 Dec 13.

Exposure to light (especially blue light)
40. http://www.health.harvard.edu/staying-healthy/blue-light-has-a-dark-side

Diabetes
41. A. S. Glicksman and R. W. Rawson, "Diabetes and altered carbohydrate metabolism in patients with cancer.," Cancer, vol. 9, no. 6, pp. 1127–34.
42. E. Giovannucci, D. M. Harlan, M. C. Archer, R. M. Bergenstal, S. M. Gapstur, L. a Habel, M. Pollak, J. G. Regensteiner, and D. Yee, "Diabetes and cancer: a consensus report.," Diabetes Care, vol. 33, no. 7, pp. 1674–85, Jul. 2010.
43. P. J. Hardefeldt, S. Edirimanne, and G. D. Eslick, "Diabetes increases the risk of breast cancer: a meta-analysis.," Endocr. Relat. Cancer, vol. 19, no. 6, pp. 793–803, Dec. 2012.
44. P. Boyle, M. Boniol, A. Koechlin, C. Robertson, F. Valentini, K. Coppens, L.-L. Fairley, T. Zheng, Y. Zhang, M. Pasterk, M. Smans, M. P. Curado, P. Mullie, S. Gandini, M. Bota, G. B. Bolli, J. Rosenstock, and P. Autier, "Diabetes and breast cancer risk: a meta-analysis.," Br. J. Cancer, vol. 107, no. 9, pp. 1608–17, Oct. 2012.
45. Centers for Disease Control and Prevention, "National diabetes fact sheet," 2011.

Thyroid cancer and breast cancer link
46. Hyun JA, Yul, H, Young AH, et al. A possible association between thyroid cancer and breast cancer. Thyroid. Dec 2015, 25(12):1330-1338.

Alcohol
47. Schütze M et al. Alcohol attributable burden of incidence of cancer in eight European countries based on results from prospective cohort study. BMJ. 2011 Apr 7;342:d1584.
48. https://www.pennmedicine.org/news/news-releases/2014/july/new-study-shows-drinking-alcoh

Triple negative breast cancer
49. Swain S. Triple-Negative Breast Cancer: Metastatic risk and role of platinum agents 2008 ASCO Clinical Science Symposium 2008. June 3, 2008.
50. Trivers KF, Lund MJ, Porter PL et al. The epidemiology of triple-negative breast cancer, including race. Cancer Causes Control 2009; 20: 1071.

Reproductive risk factors
51. Carey LA, Perou CM, Livasy CA, et al. Race, breast cancer subtypes, and survival in the Carolina Breast Cancer Study. JAMA 2006; 295:2492.
52. Phipps AI, Chlebowski RT, Prentice R, et al. Reproductive history and oral contraceptive use in relation to risk of triple-negative breast cancer. J Natl Cancer Inst 2011; 103: 470.
53. Phipps AI, Chlebowski RT, Prentice R, et al. Reproductive history and oral contraceptive use in relation to risk of triple-negative breast cancer. J Natl Cancer Inst 2011; 103: 470.
54. Anderson KN, Schwab RB, Martinez ME. Reproductive risk factors and breast cancer subtypes: a systematic review of the literature. Breast Cancer Res Treat 2014; 144: 1.
55. Pierobon M, Frenkenfeld CL. Obesity as a risk factor for triple-negative breast caners: a systematic review and meta-analysis. Breast Cancer Res Treat 2013; 137: 307.
56. Palmer JR, Viscidi E, Troester MA, et al. Parity, lactation, and breast cancer subtypes in African American women: results from the AMBER Consortium. J Natl Cancer Inst 2014; 106.

Breast cancer subtypes
57. Gonzalez-Angulo AM, Timms KM, et al. Incidence and outcome of BRCA mutations in unselected patients with triple receptor-negative breast cancer. Clin Cancer Res 2011; 17: 1082.

58. Millikan RC, Newman B, Tse CK, et al. Epidemiology of basal-like breast cancer. Breast Cancer Res Treat 2008; 109:123.

59. Parise CA, Bauer KR, Brown MM, et al. Breast cancer subtypes as defined by the estrogen receptor (ER), progesterone receptor (PR), and the human epidermal growth factor receptor 2 (HER2) among women with invasive breast cancer in California, 1999-2004. Breast J 2009; 15: 593.

Male breast cancer

60. cancer.org/cancer/breastcancerinmen/detailedguide/breast-cancer-in-men-risk factors

61. cancer.org/cancer/breastcancerinmen/detailedguide/breast-cancer-in-men-risk-factors

Exposure to radiation

62. Land CE, Tokunaga M, Koyama K et al. Incidence of female breast cancer among atomic bomb survivors. Hiroshima and Nagasaki, 1950-1990. Radiat Res 2003;;160: 707-717.

63. Preston DL, Mattsson A, Holmberg E et al. Radiation effects on breast cancer risk for young women treated for Hodgkin lymphoma. J Natl Cancer Inst 2005; 97:1428-37.

Tobacco

64. Gaudet MM, Gapstur SM, Sun J, et al. Active smoking and breast cancer risk: original cohort data and meta-analysis. J Natl Cancer Inst. 105(8):515-25, 2013.

65. Dossus L, Boutron-Ruault MC, Kaaks R, et al. for the European Prospective Investigation into Cancer and Nutrition (EPIC) cohort. Active and passive cigarette smoking and breast cancer risk: results from the EPIC cohort. Int J Cancer. 134(8):1871-88, 2014.

66. Xue F, Willett WC, Rosner BA, Hankinson SE, Michels KB. Cigarette smoking and the incidence of breast cancer. Arch Intern Med. 171(2):125-133, 2011.

67. Hamajima N, Hirose K, Tajima K, et al. for the Collaborative Group on Hormonal Factors in Breast Cancer. Alcohol, tobacco and breast cancer--collaborative reanalysis of individual data from 53 epidemiological studies, including 58,515 women with breast cancer and 95,067 women without the disease. Br J Cancer. 87(11):1234-45, 2002.

68. Macacu A, Autier P, Boniol M, Boyle P. Active and passive smoking and risk of breast cancer: a meta-analysis. Breast Cancer Res Treat. 154(2):213-24, 2015.

"Preventative" Breast Removal

69. Newman LA ed. Surgical Oncology Clinics of North America, 2014; vol 23 (3).

DES

70. Howlader N, Noone AM,, Krapcho M, et al. (eds.) SEER Cancer Statistics Review, 1975-2009 (Vintage 2009 Populations), NCI. Bethesda, MD, 2012. Retrieved April 25, 2017.

Risk Calculators

71. http://ccge.medschl.cam.ac.uk/boadicea/ Centre for Cancer Genetic Epidemiology. BOADI-CEA. Accessed March 14, 2017.

72. http://www.ems-trials.org/riskevaluation/ Accessed March 14, 2017.

73. https://www.cancer.gov/bcrisktool/ Accessed March 14, 2017.

74. http://www.yourdiseaserisk.wustl.edu/ Siteman Cancer Center. Accessed March 14, 2017.

Implementing risk reduction

75. Goss PR, Ingle JN, Pritchard K, et al: Extending aromatase-inhibitor therapy to 10 years. N Engl J Med 375:209-219, 2016.

76. Chlebowski R. Improving Breast Cancer Risk Assessment Versus Implementing Breast Cancer Prevention. J Clin Oncol, 35(7), 2017: 702-704.

77. Newman L and Petrelli N, eds. Breast cancer. Surgicl Oncology Clinics of North America 23 (3): 424-425, 2014.

Oral contraceptives

78. Collaborative Group on Hormonal Factors in Breast Cancer. Breast cancer and hormonal contraceptives: collaborative reanalysis of individual data on 53,297 women with breast cancer and 100,239 women without breast cancer from 54 epidemiological studies. Collaborative Group on Hormonal Factors in Breast Cancer. Lancet. 347:1713-27, 1996.

79. Gierisch JM, Coeytaux RR, Urrutia RP, et al. Oral contraceptive use and risk of breast, cervical, colorectal, and endometrial cancers: a systematic review. Cancer Epidemiol Biomarkers Prev. 22(11):1931-43, 2013.

Breast feeding

80. Collaborative Group on Hormonal Factors in Breast Cancer. Breast cancer and breast feeding: collaborative reanalysis of individual data from 47 epidemiological studies in 30 countries, including 50,302 women with breast cancer and 96,973 women without the disease. Lancet 20:187-95, 2002.

Hormone replacement therapy

81. Goss PE, Ingle JN, Alés-Martínez JE, et al. for the NCIC CTG MAP.3 Study Investigators. Exemestane for breast-cancer prevention in postmenopausal women. N Engl J Med. 364(25):2381-91, 2011.

82. U.S. Food and Drug Administration. Menopause and hormones: Common questions. http://www.fda.gov/ForConsumers/ByAudience/ForWomen/ucm118624.htm, 2014.

83. Holmberg L, Iverson OE, Rudenstam CM, et al., for the HABITS Study Group. Increased risk of recurrence after hormone replacement therapy in breast cancer survivors.J Natl Cancer Inst. 100(7):475-82, 2008.

84. Colditz GA, Hankinson SE, Hunter DJ, et al. The use of estrogens and progestins and the risk of breast cancer in postmenopausal women. N Engl J Med. 332: 1589-93, 1995.

85. Cancer Epidemiol Biomarkers Prev. 2005 Dec;14(12):2905-13.
Migration history, acculturation, and breast cancer risk in Hispanic women.

86. John EM1, Phipps AI, Davis A, Koo J. Cancer Epidemiol Biomarkers Prev. 2005 Dec;14(12):2905-13.Migration history, acculturation, and breast cancer risk in Hispanic women.

Worldwide - Incidence

87. https://www.wcrf.org/dietandcancer/cancer-trends/breast-cancer-statistics

88. Wingo PA, Jamison PM, Young JL, et al. "Population-based statistics for women diagnosed with inflammatory breast cancer (United States)," Cancer Causes and Control, vol. 15, no. 3, pp. 321–328, 2004.

89. Hance KW, Anderson WF, Devesa SS, et al. "Trends in inflammatory breast carcinoma incidence and survival: the surveillance, epidemiology, and end results program at the National Cancer Institute," Journal of the National Cancer Institute, vol. 97, no. 13, pp. 966–975, 2005. View at Publisher · View at Google Scholar · View at Scopus

09. Anderson WF, Schairer C, and Chen BE. "Epidemiology of inflammatory breast cancer (IBC)," Breast Disease, vol. 22, pp. 9–23, 2005.

91. Chang S, Parker SL, Pham T. "Inflammatory breast carcinoma incidence and survival: The Surveillance, Epidemiology, and End Results program of the National Cancer Institute, 1975–1992," Cancer, vol. 82, no. 12, pp. 2366–2372, 1998.

92. Stocks LH and Patterson FM, "Inflammatory carcinoma of the breast," Surgery, Gynecology & Obstetrics, vol. 143, no. 6, pp. 885–889, 1976.

93. Levine H, Steinhorn SC, L. et al. "Inflammatory breast cancer: 6. The experience of the surveillance, epidemiology, and end results (SEER) program," Journal of the National Cancer Institute, vol. 74, no. 2, pp. 291–297, 1985.

94. Jaiyesimi IA, A. Buzdar U, and Hortobagyi G, "Inflammatory breast cancer: A review," Journal of Clinical Oncology, vol. 10, no. 6, pp. 1014–1024, 1992.

95. Dawood S, Lei X, Dent R, et al. Survival of women with inflammatory breast cancer: a large population-based study. *Ann Oncol* 2014; 25(6): 1143-1151.

History

96. Bell C. A system of operative surgery founded on the basis of anatomy. Hale and Hosmer; Hartford, CT: 1816.

97. Lee BJ and Tannenbaum NE. Inflammatory carcinoma of the breast. Surg Gynecol Obstet 1924;39:580-595.

98. Treves N. Inflammatory carcinoma of the breast in the male patient. Surgery 1953;34:810-820.

99. Leitch A. Peau d'orange in acute mammary carcinoma: Its cause and diagnostic value. Lancet. 1909:1:861-863.

100. Haagensen CD. Diseases of the breast. WB Saunders; Philadelphia: 1971. 576-584; 808-814.

Age

101. Bryant T. Diseases of the breast. Cassell & Company, Limited; London, Paris, New York, and Melbourne: 1887, 186-194.

102. Anderson WF, Schairer C, Chen B, et al. Epidemiology of inflammatory breast cancer (IBC). Breast Dis 2005; 22:9-23.

103. Hance KW, Anderson WF, Devesa SS, et al. "Trends in inflammatory breast carcinoma incidence and survival: the surveillance, epidemiology, and end results program at the National Cancer Institute," Journal of the National Cancer Institute, vol. 97, no. 13, pp. 966–975, 2005.

104. Wingo PA, Jamison OM, Young JL, and P. Gargiullo, "Population-based statistics for women diagnosed with inflammatory breast cancer (United States)," Cancer Causes and Control, vol. 15, no. 3, pp. 321–328, 2004.

105. Anderson WF, Schairer C, Chen BE, et al. "Epidemiology of inflammatory breast cancer (IBC)," Breast Disease, vol. 22, pp. 9–23, 2005.

106. Chang S, Parker SL, Pham T, et al. "Inflammatory breast carcinoma incidence and survival: The Surveillance, Epidemiology, and End Results program of the National Cancer Institute, 1975–1992," Cancer, vol. 82, no. 12, pp. 2366–2372, 1998.

Reproductive factors

107. Chang S, Buzdar AU, Hursting SD. Inflammatory breast cancer and body mass index. J Clin Oncol 1998;16:3731-3735.

108. Hance KW, Anderson WF, Devesa SS et al. Trends in inflammatory breast carcinoma incidence and survival: the surveillance, epidemiology, and end results program at the National Cancer Institute. J Natl Cancer Inst 2005; 97:966.

109. Anderson WF, Schairer C, Chen BE te al. Epidemiology of inflammatory breast cancer (IBF). Breast Dis 2005-2006; 22:9.

110. Bristol IK, Woodward WA, Strom EA et al. Locoregional treatment outcomes after multimodality management of inflammatory breast cancer. Int J Radiat Oncol Biop Phys 2008; 72:474.

Other

111. Anderson WF, Schairer C, Chen BE te al. Epidemiology of inflammatory breast cancer (IBF). Breast Dis 2005-2006; 22:9.

2 image

Mammograms

1. U.S. Preventive Services Task Force. Ann Intern Med. 151(10):716-726, 2009.

2. http://www.cancer.org/cancer/breastcancer/moreinformation/breastcancerearlydetection/breast-cancer-early-detection-acs-rec

3. http://www.nccn.org/professionals/physician_gls/pdf/breast-screening.pdf

Age

4. NCI-funded Breast Cancer Surveillance Consortium (HHSN26121000031C) http://breas screening.cancer.gov/ (Accessed on November 09, 2015).

5. Fletcher SW, Elmore JG. Clinical practice. Mammographic screening for breast cancer. N Engl J Med. 2003;348:1672-1680.

6. Schonberg MA, McCarthy EP, Davis RB, et al. Breast cancer screening in women aged 80 and older: results from a national survey. J Am Geriatr Soc. 2004;52:1688-1695.

7. Schonberg MA, Ramanan RA, McCarthy EP, Marcantonio ER. Decision making and counseling around mammography screening for women aged 80 or older. J Gen Intern Med. 2006;21:979-985.

Breast Tumor Prognostic Characteristics and Biennial vs Annual Mammography, Age, and Menopausal Status

8. Miglioretti DL, Zhu W, Kerlikowske K. Breast tumor prognostic characteristics and biennial vs annual mammography, age, and menopausal status. JAMA Oncol. 2015;1(8):1069-1077.

Mammograms: Cons

9. U.S. Preventive Services Task Force. Screening for breast cancer: U.S. Preventive Services Task Force recommendation statement. Ann Intern Med. 151(10):716-726, 2009.

10. Ronckers CM, Erdmann CA, Land CE: Radiation and breast cancer: a review of current evidence. Breast Cancer Res 7 (1): 21-32, 2005.

11. Goss PE, Sierra S: Current perspectives on radiation-induced breast cancer. J Clin Oncol 16 (1): 338-47, 1998.

12. Radiology 241 (1): 55-66, 2006.

13. Bleyer A, Welch HG: N Engl J Med 367 (21): 1998-2005, 2012.

14. Jørgensen KJ, Gøtzsche PC: BMJ 339: b2587, 2009.

15. Kalager M, Zelen M, Langmark F, et al.: N Engl J Med 363 (13): 1203-10, 2010.

Breast MRI

16. American College of Radiology. ACR Practice Parameter for the Performance of Contrast-Enhanced Magnetic Resonance Imaging (MRI) of the Breast. http://www.acr.org/~/media/2a0eb 28eb59041e2825179afb72ef624.pdf. Accessed June 15, 2015.

17. Dontchos BN, DeMartini WB, Rahbar H, Peacock S, Lehman CD. Influence of Menstrual Cycle Timing on Screening Breast MRI Performance in Pre-Menopausal Women. Presented at: Radiological Society of North America (RSNA) Annual Meeting; November 25-30, 2012; Chicago, IL.

18. Saslow D et al. CA Cancer J Clin 2007;57:75-89

19. Berg WA, Zhang Z, Lehrer D, et al. for the ACRIN 6666 Investigators. Detection of breast cancer with addition of annual screening ultrasound or a single screening MRI to mammography in women with elevated breast cancer risk. JAMA. 307(13):1394-404, 2012.

20. Pinsky RW, Helvie MA. Mammographic breast density: effect on imaging and breast cancer risk. J Natl Compr Canc Netw. 8(10):1157-64, 2010.
21. Tagliafico AS, et al. Adjuvant screening with tomosynthesis or ultrasound in women with mammography-negative dense breasts: Interim report of a prospective comparative trial. J Clin Oncol 34: 1883-88 (16), 2016.
22. O'Flynn EA, Ledger AE, deSouza NM. Alternative screening for dense breasts: MRI. AJR Am J Roentgenol. 204(2):W141-9, 2015.

Ultrasound
23. Berg WA, Zhang Z, Lehrer D, et al. for the ACRIN 6666 Investigators. Detection of breast cancer with addition of annual screening ultrasound or a single screening MRI to mammography in women with elevated breast cancer risk. JAMA. 307(13):1394-404, 2012.
24. Scheel JR, Lee JM, Sprague BL, Lee CI, Lehman CD. Screening ultrasound as an adjunct to mammography in women with mammographically dense breasts. Am J Obstet Gynecol. 212(1):9-17. 2015.

Tomosynthesis
25. Skaane P, Bandos AI, Gullien R, et al. Comparison of digital mammography alone and digital mammography plus tomosynthesis in a population-based screening program. Radiology. 267(1):47-56, 2013.
26. Ciatto S, Houssami N, Bernardi D, et al. Integration of 3D digital mammography with tomosynthesis for population breast-cancer screening (STORM): a prospective comparison study. Lancet Oncol. S1470-2045(13)70134-7, 2013.
27. Friedewald SM, Rafferty EA, Rose SL, et al. Breast cancer screening using tomosynthesis in combination with digital mammography. JAMA. 311(24):2499-2507, 2014.
28.http://www.cancer.org/cancer/news/news/breast-cancer-screening-with-3-d-technology-finds-more-cancers
25. http://www.massgeneral.org/imaging/services/3D_mammography_tomosynthesis.aspx
High-risk: Screening
29. American Cancer Society. Mammogram reports – BI-RADS.
30. U.S. Preventive Services Task Force. Screening for breast cancer: U.S. Preventive Services Task Force recommendation statement. Ann Intern Med. 151(10):716-726, 2009.
31. http://www.facingourrisk.org/understanding-brca-and-hboc/publications/documents/Surveillance%20Flyer%207.16.14.pdf

Molecular imaging
32. Hendrick RE. Radiation doses and cancer risks from breast imaging studies. Radiology. 257(1):246-53, 2010.

Clinical breast exam
33. Fenton JJ, Rolnick SJ, Harris EL, et al.: Specificity of clinical breast examination in community practice. J Gen Intern Med 22 (3): 332-7, 2007.

Self-exam
34. Thomas DB, Gao DL, Ray RM, et al.: Randomized trial of breast self-examination in Shanghai: final results. J Natl Cancer Inst 94 (19): 1445-57, 2002.
35. Semiglazov VF, Manikhas AG, Moiseenko VM, et al.: [Results of a prospective randomized investigation [Russia (St.Petersburg)/WHO] to evaluate the significance of self-examination for the early detection of breast cancer]. Vopr Onkol 49 (4): 434-41, 2003.

Thermography
36. Lee CI and Elmore JC. Chap 11. Breast Cancer Screening, in Harris JR, Lippman ME, Morrow M, Osborne CK. Diseases of the Breast, 5th edition. Lippincott Williams and Wilkins, 2014.
37. http://www.fda.gov/NewsEvents/Newsroom/PressAnnouncements/ucm257633.htm

Breast density; high risk imaging
38. Gierach GL, Ichikawa L, Kerlikowske K, et al. Relationship between mammographic density and breast cancer death in the Breast Cancer Surveilance Consortiu. J Natl Cancer Inst 2012; 104(16):1218-27.
39. https://www.breastcancer.org/symptoms/testing/types/mri/screening

Fact box
40. Gøtzsche PC, Jørgensen KJ (2013). Cochrane Database of Systematic Reviews (6): CD001877.pub5.
41. https://www.harding-cancer.mpg.de/en/health-information/facts-boxes/mammography

Inflammatory breast cancer
42. http://www.cancer.net/cancer-types/breast-cancer-inflammatory/statistics
43. Chow CK. Imaging in inflammatory breast carcinoma. Breast Dis 2005-2006;22:45–54.
44. Tardivon AA, Viala J, Corvellec Rudelli A, Guinebretiere JM, Vanel D. Mammographic patterns of inflammatory breast carcinoma: a retrospective study of 92 cases. Eur J Radiol 1997;24(2):124–130.

3 biopsy

1. Kleer CG, van Golem KL, et al. Molecular biology of breast cancer metastasis. Inflammatory breast cancer: clinical syndrome and molecular determinants. Breast Cancer Res 2000; 2(6):423.
2. Somle G, Frankel P, et al. Prognostic indicators and survival in patients with stage IIIB inflammatory breast carcinoma after dose-intense chemotherapy. J Clin Onol 2004;22(10):1839-48.

4 pathology

Invasive ductal cancer
1. Li CI, Uribe DJ, Daling JR. Clinical characteristics of different histologic types of breast cancer. Br J Cancer 2005; 93: 1046.
2. Ménard S, Tagliabue E, Campiglio M, Pupa SM. J Cell Physiol. 2000;182:150-162.
3. Sergina NV, Rausch M, Wang D, et al. Nature. 2007;445:437-441.
61. http://www.choosingwisely.org/societies/american-society-of-clinical-oncology/
4. https://cancerstaging.org/references-tools/quickreferences/Documents/BreastMedium.pdf

HER2
5. Slamon DJ, Godolphin W, Jones LA, et al. Science. 1989;244:707-712.
6. Sliwkowski MX. In: Harris JR, Lippman ME, Morrow M, Osborne CK, eds. Diseases of the Breast. 3rd ed. Philadelphia, PA: Lippincott Williams & Wilkins; 2004:415-426.
7. Ménard S, Tagliabue E, Campiglio M, Pupa SM. Role of HER2 gene overexpression in breast carcinoma. J Cell Physiol. 2000;182:150-162.

8. http://ww5.komen.org/BreastCancer/SubtypesofBreastCancer.html#sthash.qOuPw8j5.dpuf. Accessed April 28, 2019.
9. Paradise A, Tommasi S, Brandi M, et al. Cell kinetics and hormonal receptor status in inflammatory breast carcinoma. Comparison with locally advanced disease. Cancer 1989; 1:64(9). 1922-1927.

Inflammatory breast cancer
10. Tai P, Yu E, Shiels R et al. Short- and long-term causes-specific survival of patients with inflammatory breast cancer. BMC Cancer 2005: 5:137.

5 stage

6 prognosis

7 management: overview

1. Matro, JM, Li T, Cristofanilli M et al. Inflammatory breast cancer management in the national comprehensive cancer network: the disease, recurrence pattern, and outcome. Clin Breast Cancer 2015;15:1.
2. WalsheJM, Swain SM. Clinical aspects of inflammatory breast cancer. Breast Dis 2005-2006;22:35.
3. Bauer RL, Busch E, Levine E et al. Therapy for inflammatory breast cancer: impact of doxorubicin-based therapy. Ann Surg Oncol 1995; 2:288.
4. Cristofanilli M, Buzdar AU, Sneige N et al. Paclitaxel in the multimodality treatment for inflammatory breast carcinoma. Cancer 2001; 92:1775.
5. Brzezinska M, Williams LJ, Thomas J et al. Outcomes of patients with inflammatory breast cancer treated by breast-conserving surgery Breast Cancer Res Treat 2016; 160:387.
6. StearnsV, Ewing CA, Slack R, et al. Sentinel lymphadenectomy after neoadjuvant chemotherapy for breast cancer may reliably represent the axilla except for inflammatory breast cancer. Ann Surg Oncol 2002; 9:235.
7. Chin PL, Andersen JS, Somlo G, et al. Esthetic reconstruction after mastectomy for inflammatory breast cancer: is it worthwhile? J Am Coll Surg 2000; 190:304.
8. Motwani SB, Strom EA, Schechter NR, et al. The impact of immediate breast reconstruction on the technical delivery of postmastectomy radiotherapy. Int J Radiat Oncol Biol Phys 2006; 66:76.
9. Liauw SL, Benda RK, Morris CG, et al. Locoregional irradiation for inflammatory breast cancer: effectiveness of dose escalation in decreasing recurrence. Int J Radiat Oncol Biol Phys 2000; 47:1191.
10. Bristol IJ, Woodward WA, Strom EA, et al. Locoregional treatment outcomes after multimodality management of inflammatory breast cancer Int J Radiat Oncol Biol Phys 2008; 72:474.

11. Li BD, Sicard MA, Ampil F, et al. Trimodal therapy for inflammatory breast cancer: a surgeon's perspective. Oncology 2010;79(1-2):3-12.

12. Masuda H, Brewer TM, Liu DD, et al. Long-term treatment efficacy in primary inflammatory breast cancer by hormonal receptor- and HER2-defined subtypes. Annals of Oncology 2014; 25(2):384-91. [

13. Merajver SD, Sabel MS. Inflammatory breast cancer. In: Harris JR, Lippman ME, Morrow M, Osborne CK, editors. Diseases of the Breast. 3rd ed. Philadelphia: Lippincott Williams and Wilkins, 2004.

14. Ries LAG, Young JL, Keel GE, et al (editors). SEER Survival Monograph: Cancer Survival Among Adults: U.S. SEER Program, 1988-2001, Patient and Tumor Characteristics. Bethesda, MD: NCI SEER Program; 2007. NIH Pub. No. 07-6215.

15. Robertson FM, Bondy M, Yang W, et al. Inflammatory breast cancer: the disease, the biology, the treatment. CA: A Cancer Journal for Clinicians 2010; 60(6):351-375.

16. Rueth NM, Lin HY, Bedrosian I, et al. Underuse of trimodality treatment affects survival for patients with inflammatory breast cancer: an analysis of treatment and survival trends from the National Cancer Database. Journal of Clinical Oncology 2014; 32(19):2018-24.

17. Schairer C, Li Y, Frawley P, Graubard BI, et al. Risk factors for inflammatory breast cancer and other invasive breast cancers. Journal of the National Cancer Institute 2013; 105(18):1373-1384.

18. Tsai CJ, Li J, Gonzalez-Angulo AM, et al. Outcomes after multidisciplinary treatment of inflammatory breast cancer in the era of neoadjuvant HER2-directed therapy. American Journal of Clinical Oncology 2015; 38(3):242-247.

19. Van Laere SJ, Ueno NT, Finetti P, et al. Uncovering the molecular secrets of inflammatory breast cancer biology: an integrated analysis of three distinct affymetrix gene expression datasets. Clinical Cancer Research 2013; 19(17):4685-96. [PubMed Abstract]

20. Yamauchi H, Ueno NT. Targeted therapy in inflammatory breast cancer. Cancer 2010; 116(11 Suppl):2758-9. [PubMed Abstract]

21. Yamauchi H, Woodward WA, Valero V, et al. Inflammatory breast cancer: what we know and what we need to learn. The Oncologist 2012; 17(7):891-9.

Chemotherapy

22. Fan C, Oh DS, Wessels L, et al. Concordance among gene-expression-based predictors for breast cancer. N Engl J Med. 355(6):560-9, 2006.

23. Koboldt DC, Fulton RS, McLellan MD, et al. for the Cancer Genome Atlas Network. Comprehensive molecular portraits of human breast tumours. Nature. 490(7418):61-70, 2012.

24. Kohler BA, Sherman RL, Howlader N, et al. Annual report to the nation on the status of cancer, 1975-2011, featuring incidence of breast cancer subtypes by race/ethnicity, poverty, and state. J Natl Cancer Inst. 107(6), 2015.

Side effects

4. Lagos R et al. Towards diagnostic imaging of ChemoBrain phenomenon" RSNA 2012; Abstract LL-MIS-TU2A.

8 chemo

5. http://www.webmd.com/ovarian-cancer/features/appearance-during-chemo patterns of recurrence. Clin Cancer Res 2--7;13(15 Pt 1):4429-34.

6. Janelsins M, Heckler C, Peppone L et al. Cognitive complaints in survivors of breast cancer after chemotherapy compared with age-matched controls: An analysis from a nationwide, multi-center, prospective longitudinal study J Clin Oncol 35: 506-514.

Pregnancy after treatment: Safe?

7. Valachis A, Tsali L, Pesce LL et al. Safety of pregnancy after primary breast carcinoma in young women: a meta-analysis to overcome bias of healthy mother effect tudies. Obstet Gynecol Surg 2010; 65:786.

8. Azim HA Jr, Sabtoro L, Pavlidis N et al. Safety of pregnancy following breast cancer diagnosis: a meta-analysis of 14 studies. Eur J Cancer 2011;47:74.

Herceptin

9. Perez EA, Romond EH, Suman VJ et al. Trastazumab plus adjuvant chemotherapy for human epidermal growth factor receptor 2-positive breast cancer: planned joint analysis of overall survival from NSABP B-31 and NCCTG N9831: J Clin Oncol 2014; 32:3744.

10. Gianni L, Dafni U, Gelber RD et al. Treatment with trastazumab for 1 year after adjuvant chemotherapy in patients with HER2-positive early breast cancer: a 4-year follow-up of a ran-domised controlled trial. Lancet Oncol 2011; 12:236.

11. Goldhirsch A, Gelber RD, Oiccart-Gebhart MJ et al. 2 years versus 1 year of adjuvant trasta-zumab for HER2-positive breast cancer (HERA): an open-label, randomised controlled trial. Lancet 2013; 14:741.

12. Pivot X, Romieu G, Debled M et al. 6 months versus 12 months of adjuvant trastazumab for HER2-positive early breast cancer (PHARE): a randomised phase 3 trial. Lancet Oncol 2013; 14:741.

13. Pivot X, Suter T, Nabholtz JM et al. Cardiac toxicity events in the PHARE trial, an adjuvant trastazumab randomised phase III study. Eur J Cancer 2015;51:1660.

14. Perez EA, Romond EH, Suman VJ et al. Four-year follow-up of trastazumab plus adjuvant chemotherapy for operable human epidermal growth factor receptor 2-positive breast cancer: joint analysis of data from NCCTG N9831 and NSABP B-31. J Clin Oncol 2011;29:336.

15, Gianni L, Eiermann W, Semiglazov V et al. Neoadjuvant and adjuvant trastazumab in pa-tients with HER2-positive locally advanced breast cancer (NOAH): follow-up of a randomized controlled superiority trial and parallel HER2-negative cohort. Lancet Oncology 2014; 15(6): 640-647.

CAR-T cell therapy for brain metastases

15. https://www.healio.com/hematology-oncology/breast-cancer/news/online/%7B68f57e59-2188-475c-af92-e2daa99b5fb3%7D/trial-to-assess-car-t-cell-therapy-for-her2-pos-itive-metastatic-breast-cancer?utm_source=selligent&utm_medium=email&utm_campaign=hematology%20oncology%20news&m_bt=1690795913719

16. Piccart-Gebhart MJ, Procter M, Leyland-Jones B et al. Trastazumab after adjuvant chemo-therapy in HER2-positive breast cancer. N Engl J Med 2005;353:1659.

17. lamon D Eiermann W, Robert N et al. Adjuvant trastazumab in HER2-positive breast cancer. N Eng J Med 2011;365:1273.

18. NCCN Clinical Practice Guidelines in Oncology (NCCN Guidelines). Breast Cancer (ver-sion 2.2016. https://www.nccn.org/professionals/physician_gls/pdf/breast.pdf (Accessed on June 12, 2016).

19. Moja L, Tagliabue L, Balduzzu S et al. Trastazumab containing regiment for early breast cancer. Cochrane Database Syst Rev 2012:4:CD006243.

Scalp cooling for chemotherapy-induced hair loss
20. Rugo H et al.: 2016 MASCC/ISOO International Symposium. Presented June 23, 2016.

Triple negative breast cancer
21. University of Colorado Anschutz Medical Campus. "Finally, targeted therapies for triple-negative breast cancer: Promising clinical trials of IMMU-132, vantictumab and atezolizumab against TNBC." ScienceDaily. ScienceDaily, 4 June 2016.
22. Dent R, Trudeau M, Pritchard KI et al. Triple-negative breast cancer; Clinical features and
23. National Comprehensive Cancer Network (NCCN). NCCN Clinical practice guidelines in oncology: Breast cancer V.1.2016. http://www.nccn.org/, 2016.

Fertility
24. National Comprehensive Cancer Network (NCCN). NCCN Clinical practice guidelines in oncology: Breast cancer V.1.2016. http://www.nccn.org/, 2016.
25. Jeruss JS, Woodruff TK. Preservation of fertility in patients with cancer. N Engl J Med. 360(9):902-11, 2009.
26. American College of Obstetricians and Gynecologists' Committee on Gynecologic Practice: Committee Opinion No. 584: oocyte cryopreservation. Obstet Gynecol. 123(1):221-2, 2014.
27. Lambertini M, Boni L, Michelotti A, et al. for the GIM Study Group. Ovarian suppression with triptorelin during adjuvant breast cancer chemotherapy and long-term ovarian function, pregnancies, and disease-free survival: a randomized clinical trial. JAMA. 314(24):2632-40, 2015.
28. Munhoz RR, Pereira AA, Sasse AD, et al. Gonadotropin-releasing hormone agonists for ovarian function preservation in premenopausal women undergoing chemotherapy for early-stage breast cancer: a systematic review and meta-analysis. JAMA Oncol. 2(1):65-73, 2016.

Residual cancer after neoadjuvant chemotherapy
29. Masuda N, Lee S, Ohtani, S et al. Adjuvant capecitabine for breast cancer after preoperative chemotherapy. N Engl J Med 2017; 376:2147-2159.

Surgery: BRCA
30. Howlader N, Noone AM, Krapcho M, et al. (eds). SEER Cancer Statistics Review, 1975-2011, National Cancer Institute. Bethesda, MD, http://seer.cancer.gov/csr/1975_2011/ , based on November 2013 SEER data submission, posted to the SEER web site, April 2014.

9 surgery

10 radiation

Radiation therapy: Dose escalation
1. Liao Z, Strom EA, Buzdar AU, et al. Locoregional irradiation for inflammatory breast cancer: effectiveness of dose escalation in decreasing recurrence. Int J Radiat Oncol Biol Phys 2000;47(5):1191.

Radiation therapy: Modern techniques reduce complications

2. Darby SC, Ewertz M, McGale P et al. Risk of ischemic heart disease in women after radiotherapy or breast cancer N Engl J Med 2013; 368:987-998.

3. Schaapveld M, Visser O, Louwman M et al. Risk of new primary nonbreast cancers after breast cancer treatment: A Dutch population-based study. J Clin Oncol 2008;26(8):1239-1246.

4. Management of symptomatic vulvovaginal atrophy: 2013 position statement of The North American Menopause Society. Menopause 2013; Sep:20(9):888-902; quiz 903-904.

5. Meric F, Bucholz TA, Mirza NQ et al. Long-term complications associated with breast-conservation surgery and radiotherapy. Ann Surg Oncol 2002;9(6):543.

6. Whelan TJ, Olivotto I, Ackerman I, et al. NCIC-CTG MA.20: an intergroup trial of regional nodal irradiation in early breast cancer. Program and abstracts of the 2011 American Society of Clinical Oncology Annual Meeting; June 3-7, 2011; Chicago, Illinois. Abstract LBA1003.

Radiation therapy: Risk of causing cancer

7. Rombouts, AJM; Huising J, Hugen, N et. al. Assessment of Radiotherapy-Associated Angiosarcoma After Breast Cancer Treatment in a Dutch Population-Based Study. JAMA Oncol. Published online January 24, 2019. doi:10.1001/jamaoncol.2018.6643.

11 endocrine

Endocrine therapy

1. Francis PA Regan MM, Fleming GF et al. Adjuvant ovarian suppression in premenopausal breast cancer. N Engl J Med 2015; 372:436.

2. LHRH-agonists in Early Breast Cancer Overview group. Cuzick J, Ambroisine L, et al. Use of luteinising-hormone-releasing hormone agonists as adjuvant treatment in premenopausal patients with hormone-receptor-positive breast cancer: a meta-analysis of individual patient data from randomised adjuvant trials. Lancet 2007; 369:1711.

3. Tevaarwerk AJ, Wang M, Zhao F, et al. Phase III comparison of tamoxifen versus tamoxifen plus ovarian function suppression in premenopausal women with node-negative, hormone receptor-positive breast cancer (E-3193, INT-0142): a trial of the Eastern Cooperative Oncology Group. J Clin Oncol 2014; 32:3948.

4. Steams V, Ullmer L, Lopez JF, et al. Hot flushes. Lancet 2002;360(9348; 1851.

5. Day R. Quality of life and tamoxifen in a breast cancer prevention trial: a summary of findings from the NSABP P-1 study. National Surgical Adjuvant Breast and Bowel Project. Ann NY Acad Sci 2001;949:143.

6. Jin Y, Hayes DF, Robarge JD et al. Estrogen receptor genotypes influence hot flash prevalence and composite score before and after tamoxifen therapy. J Clin Oncol 2008;26(36):5849.

7. Davies C, Godwin J, Gray R et al. Relevance of breast cancer hormone receptors and other factors to the efficacy of adjuvant tamoxifen: patient-level meta-analysis of randomised trials. Lancet 2011;378(9793):771.

8. Fisher B, Constatino JP, Wikerham DL. Tamoxifen for prevention of breast cancer: report of the National Surgical Adjuvant Breast and Bowel Project P-1 Study. J Natl Cancer Inst 1998; 90:1371-88.

9. Curtis RE, Freedman DM, Sherman ME, Fraumeni JF Jr. Risk of malignant mixed mullerian tumors after tamoxifen therapy for breast cancer. J Natl Cancer Inst 2004;96(1):70.

10. Braithwaite RS, Chlebowski RT, Lau J, et al. Meta-analysis of vascular and neoplastic events associated with tamoxifen. J Gen Intern Med 2003;18(11):937.

11. Reis SE, Constantino JP, Wickerham DL et al. Cardopvascular effects of tamoxifen in women with and without heart disease: breast cancer prevention trial. National Surgical Adjuvant Breast and Bowel Project Breast Cancer Prevention Trial Investigators. J Natl Cancer Inst 2001;93(1):16.

12. Fisher B, Constantino JP, Wickerham DL et al. Tamoxifen for the prevention of breast cancer: current status of the National Surgical Adjuvant Breast and Bowel Project P-1 study. J Natl Cancer Inst 2005;97(22):1652.

13. Rastelli AL, Taylor ME, Gao F, Armamento-Villareal R, Jamalabadi-Majidi S, Napoli N, Ellis MJ. Vitamin D and aromatase inhibitor-induced musculoskeletal symptoms (AIMSS): a phase II, double-blind, placebo-controlled, randomized trial. Breast Cancer Research and Treatment. Online June 2011.

14. Gianni L, Panzini I, Li S et al. Ocular toxicity during adjuvant chemoendocrine therapy for early breast cancer: results from the International Breast Cancer Study Group trials. Cancer 2006; 106(3):505.

15. Bradbury BD, Lash TL, Kaye JA et al. Tamoxifen and cataracts: a null association. Breast Cancer Res Treat 2004;87(2):189.

16. Pierce LJ, Hutchins LF, Green SR et al. Sequencing of tamoxifen and radiotherapy after breast-conserving surgery in early breast cancer. J Clin Oncol 2005;23:24.

17. Early Breast Cancer Trialists' Collaborative Group (EBCTCG), DowsettM, Forbes JF et al. Aromatase inhibitors versus tamoxifen in early breast cancer: patient-level meta-analysis of the randomised trials. Lancet 2015;386:1341.

18. Kidwell KM, Harte SE, Hayes DF et al. Patient-reported symptoms and discontinuation of adjuvant aromatase inhibitor therapy. Cancer 2014; 120:2403.

19. Amir E, Seruga B, Niraula S et al. Toxicity of adjuvant endocrine therapy in postmenopausal breast cancer patients; a systematic review and meta-analysis. J Natl Cancer Inst 2011;103:1299.

20. Ahn PH, Vu HT, Lannin D et al. Sequence of radiotherapy with tamoxifen in conservatively managed breast cancer does not affect local relapse rates. J Clin Oncol 2005;23:17.

Hormone receptors
21. http://www.nature.com/nchembio/journal/v2/n4/fig_tab/nchembio0406-175_F1.html

Aromatase inhibitors and pre-menopausal women
22. Pagani O, Regan MM, Walley BA, et al. for the TEXT and SOFT Investigators and the International Breast Cancer Study Group. Adjuvant exemestane with ovarian suppression in premenopausal breast cancer. N Engl J Med. 371(2):107-18, 2014.

Vaginal dryness
23. Runowicz CD et al. American Cancer Society/American Society of Clinical Oncology Breast Cancer Survivorship Guideline. J Clin Oncol 2016;34(6):611.

12 distant spread

Cancer cells travel in gangs

1. https://www.fredhutch.org/en/news/releases/2016/02/shedding-new-light-on-breast-cancer-metastasis.html

2. PNAS 2016; published ahead of print February 1, 2016, doi:10.1073/pnas.1508541113.

Coping & prognosis

3. https://www.bcna.org.au/secondary-breast-cancer/finding-out-your-cancer-has-spread/

4. Brain K, Willams B, Iredale R et al. Psychological distress in men with breast cancer. J Clin Oncol 2006;24:95.

5. Lobbezoo DJ, van Kampen RJ, Voogd AC, et al. Prognosis of metastatic breast cancer: are there differences between patients with de novo and recurrent metastatic breast cancer? Br J Cancer. 112(9):1445-51, 2015.

6. Lippman ME. Chapter 74: Management summary for the care of patients with metastatic breast cancer, in Harris JR, Lippman ME, Morrow M, Osborne CK. Diseases of the Breast, 5th edition. Lippincott Williams and Wilkins, 2014.

7. Gennari A, Conte P, Rosso R, et al. Survival of metastatic breast carcinoma patients over a 20-year period: a retrospective analysis based on individual patient data from six consecutive studies. Cancer 2005;104(8):1742.

8. Greenberg PA, Hortobagyi GN, Smith TL, et al. Long-term follow-up of patients with complete remission following combination chemotherapy for metastatic breast cancer. J Clin Oncol 1996;14(8):2197.

9. Kelly BE, Soon YY, Tattersall MH, Stockler MR. How long have I got? Estimating typical, best-case, and worst-case scenarios for patients starting first-line chemotherapy for metastatic breast cancer: a systematic review of recent randomized trials. J Clin Oncol 2011;29(4):456.

10. Stockler M, Wilcken NR, Ghersi D, and Simes RJ. Systematic review of chemotherapy and endocrine therapy in metastatic breast cancer. Cancer Treat Rev 2000;26(3):151.

11. Swenerton KD, Legha SS, Smith T, et al. Prognostic factors in metastatic breast cancer treated with combination chemotherapy. Cancer Res 1979;39(5):1552.

12. Yamamoto N, Watanabe T, Katsumata N, et al. Construction and validation of a practical prognostic index for patients with metastatic breast cancer. J Clin Oncol 1998;16(7):2401.

13. Clark GM, Sledge GW Jr, Osborne CK, et al. Survival from first recurrence: relative importance of prognostic factors in 1,015 breast cancer patients. J Clin Oncol 1987;5(1):55.

14. Leivonen MK, Kalima TC. Prognostic factors associated with survival after breast cancer recurrence. Acta Oncol 1991;30(5):583.

15. Wilcken N, Hornbuckle J, Ghersi D. Chemotherapy alone versus endocrine therapy alone for metastatic breast cancer. Cochrane Database Syst Rev. 2003;2:CD002747.

16. Johnston SRD, Schiavon G. Treatment algorithms for hormone receptor-positive advanced breast cancer: going forward in endocrine therapy – overcoming resistance and introducing new agents. Am Soc Clin Oncol Educ Book. 2013;2013:e28.

17. Mauriac L, Romieu G, Bines J. Activity of fulvestrant versus exemestane in advanced breast cancer patients with or without visceral metastases: data from the EFECT trial. Breast Cancer Res Treat. 2009;117(1):69–75.

Predicting response

19. Swenerton KD, Legha SS, Smith T et al. Prognostic factors in metastatic breast cancer treated with combination chemotherapy. Cancer Res 1979;39:1552.

20. Ahmann DL, Schaid DJ, Ingle JN, et al. A randomized trial of cyclophosphamide, doxorubicin, and prednisone versus cyclophosphamide, 5-fluorouracil, and prednisone in patients with metastatic breast cancer. Am J Clin Oncol 1991; 14:179.

21. White J, Kearins O, Dodwell D, et al. Male breast carcinoma: increased awareness needed. Breast Cancer Res 2011; 13(5):219.

22. Siegel R, Ward E, Brawley O, Jemal A. Cancer statistics, 2011: the impact of eliminating socioeconomic and racial disparities on premature cancer deaths. CA Cancer J Clin 2011;61(4);212.

23. Hortobagyi GN, Smith TL, Legha SS et al. Multivariate analysis of prognostic factors in metastatic breast cancer. J Clin Oncol 1983;776.

Work-up

24. https://www.nccn.org/professionals/physician_gls/pdf/breast.pdf

Bone-protecting drugs

25. Lipton, A, Fizazi, K, Stopeck, AT. Superiority of denosumab to zoledronic acid for prevention of skeletal-related events: a combined analysis of 3 pivotal, randomised, phase 3 trials. European Journal of Cancer 1990;48 (16): 3082–92.

26. Rosen LS, Gordon D, Kaminski M, et al. Zoledronic acid versus pamidronate in the treatment of skeletal metastases in patients with breast cancer or osteolytic lesions of multiple myeloma: a phase III, double-blind, comparative trial. Cancer J 2001;7:377-387.

27. Rosen LS, Gordon DH, Dugan W, et al. Zoledronic acid is superior to pamidronate for the treatment of bone metastases in breast carcinoma patients with at least one osteolytic lesion. Cancer 2004;100:36-43.

28. Gralow J, Barlow WE, Paterson AHG, et al. Phase III trial of bisphosphonates as adjuvant therapy in primary breast cancer: SWOG/Alliance/ECOG-ACRIN/NCIC Clinical Trials Group/NRG Oncology study S0307. J Clin Oncol 33, 2015 (suppl; abstr 503).

29. Aapro M, Abrahamsson PA, Body JJ, et al. Guidance on the use of bisphosphonates in solid tumours: recommendations of an international expert panel. Ann Oncol. 19(3):420-32, 2008.

30. Rathbone EJ, Brown JE, Marshall HC, et al. Osteonecrosis of the jaw and oral health-related quality of life after adjuvant zoledronic acid: an adjuvant zoledronic acid to reduce recurrence trial subprotocol (BIG01/04). J Clin Oncol. 31(21):2685-91, 2013.

Spinal cord compression

31. https://en.wikipedia.org/wiki/Spinal_cord_compression#/media/File:Diagram_showing_a_tumour_causing_spinal_cord_compression_CRUK_081.svg

Reducing harm from whole brain radiotherapy

32. Day J, Zienius K, Gehring K et al. Interventions for preventing and ameliorating cognitive deficits in adults treated with cranial irradiation. Cochrane Database Syst Rev 2014; CD011335.

33. Brown OR, Pugh S, Laack NN et al. Memantine for the prevention of cognitive dysfunction in patients receiving whole-brain radiotherapy: a randomized, placebo-controlled trial. Neuro Oncol 2013; 15:1429.

34. Eichenbaum H, Cohen NJ (1993). Memory, Amnesia, and the Hippocampal System. MIT Press.

35. Squire, LR; Schacter DL (2002). The Neuropsychology of Memory. Guilford Press.

Breast cancer cells masquerade as neurons to sneak into the brain

36. PNAS, DOI: 10.1073/pnas.1322098111

Brain metastases treatment

37. Patchell RA, Tibbs PA, Regine WF, et al. Postoperative radiotherapy in the treatment of single metastases to the brain: a randomized trial. JAMA 1998;280:1485-1489.

38. Paek SH, Audu PB, Sperling MR, et al. Reevaluation of surgery for the treatment of brain metastases: review of 208 patients with single or multiple brain metastases treated at one institution with modern neurosurgical techniques. Neurosurgery 2005;56:1021-1034.

39. Stark AM, Tscheslog H, Buhl R, et al. Surgical treatment for brain metastases: prognostic factors and survival in 177 patients. Neurosurg Rev 2005;28:115-119.

40. Karlsson B, Hanssens P, Wolff R, et al. Thirty years' experience with Gamma Knife surgery for metastases to the brain. J Neurosurg 2009;111:449-457.

41. Kased N, Binder DK, McDermott MW, et al. Gamma Knife radiosurgery for brain metastases from primary breast cancer. Int J Radiat Oncol Biol Phys 2009;75:1132-1140.

42. Bindal RK, Sawaya R, Leavens ME et al. Reoperation for recurrent metastatic brain tumors. J Neurosurg 1995; 83:600.

43. https://en.m.wikipedia.org/wiki/Breast_cancer#/media/File%3ADiagram_showing_stage_4_breast_cancer_CRUK_228.svg

44. http://www.choosingwisely.org/societies/american-society-for-radiation-oncology/

Radiosurgery

45. Aoyama H, Shirato H, Tago M, et al. Stereotactic radiosurgery plus whole-brain radiation therapy vs stereotactic radiosurgery alone for treatment of brain metastases: a randomized controlled trial. JAMA 2006;295:2483-2491.

46. Tsao M, Xu W, Sahgal A. A meta-analysis evaluating stereotactic radiosurgery, whole-brain radiotherapy, or both for patients presenting with a limited number of brain metastases. Cancer 212;118:2486- 2493.

47. Cooper JS, Steinfeld AD, Lerch IA. Cerebral metastases: value of reirradiation in selected patients. Radiology 1990;174:883-885.

48. Sadikov E, Bezjak A, Yi QL, et al. Value of whole brain re- irradiation for brain metastases--single centre experience. Clin Oncol (R Coll Radiol) 2007;19:532-538.

Re-recurrence in brain: Treatment

49. Wong WW, Schild SE, Sawyer TE, Shaw EG. Analysis of outcome in patients reirradiated for brain metastases. Int J Radiat Oncol Biol Phys 1996;34:585-590.

50. Chao ST, Barnett GH, Vogelbaum MA et al. Salvage stereotactic radiosurgery effectively treats recurrences from whole-brain radiation therapy. Cancer 2008; 113:2195.

14 after

Young

1. https://www.cdc.gov/cancer/breast/young_women/index.htm

2. Tai P, Yu E, Shiels R, et al. Short- and long-term cause-specific survival of patients with inflammatory breast cancer. BMC Cancer 2005; 5:137.

3. Antoniou A, Pharoah PD, Narod S, et al. Average risks of breast and ovarian cancer associated with BRCA1 or BRCA2 mutations detected in case series unselected for family history: A combined analysis of 22 studies. American Journal of Human Genetics 2003; 72(5):1117–1130.

4. https://www.cdc.gov/cancer/breast/young_women/index.htm

5. Hance KW, Anderson WF, Devesa SS et al. Trends in inflammatory breast carcinoma incidence and survival: the surveillance, epidemiology, and end results program at the National Cancer Institute. J Natl Cancer Inst 2005; 97:966.

6. https://www.cdc.gov/cancer/breast/young_women/index.htm

Lymphedema

7. Ozaslan C. Lymphedema after treatment of breast cancer. *Am J Surg* 2004; 187(1):69-72.
8. Erickson VS, Pearson ML, Ganz PA et al. Arm edema in breast cancer patients. J Natl Cancer Inst 2001;93(2):96.
9. McDuff SGR, Mina AI, Brunelle CL et al. Timing of lymphedema after treatment of breast cancer: when are patients most at risk? Int J Radiat Oncol Biol Phys 2019103(1):62.
10. Bloomquist K, Oturai P, Steele ML et al. Heavy-load lifting: Acute response in breast cacer survivors at risk for lymphedema. Med Sci Sports Exer 2018;50(2):187.
11. Moseley Al, Loller NB. Exercise for limb edema: Evidence that it is beneficial. J Lymphoedema 2008;3:51.
12. Schmitz KH, Ahmed Rl, Troxel A, et al. Weight lifting in women with breast-cancer-related lymphedema. N Engl J Med 2009;361(7):664.
13. Ahmed RL, Thomas W, Yee D, Schmitz KH. Randomized controlled trial of weight training and lymphedema in breast cancer survivors. J Clin Oncol 2006;24(18):2765.
14. Ezzo J, Manheimer E, McNeely ML, et al. Manual lymphatic drainage for lymphedema following breast cancer treatment. Cochrane Database Syst Rev 2015.
15. Didem K, Ufuk YS, and Sumre A. The comparison of two different physiotherapy methods in treatment of lymphedema after breast surgery. Breast Cancer Res Treat 2005;93(1):49.
16. Dayes IS, Whelan TJ, Julian JA et al. Randomized trial of decongestive lymphatic drainage for the treatment of lymphedema in women with breast cancer. J Clin Oncol 2013;31(30):3758-63.
17. DiSipio T, Rye S, Newman B, Hayes S. Incidence of unilateral arm lymphoedema after breast cancer: a systematic review and meta-analysis. Lancet Oncol 2013;14(6):500.

Follow-up

18. GLOBOCON 2008 Update http:www.iarc.fr/en/media-centre/iarcnews/2011/globocon2008-prev.php
19. DeSantis CE, Lin CC, Mariotto AB et al. Cancer treatment and survivorship statistis, 2014. CA Cancer J Clin 2014; 64(4): 252.
20.Kwan ML, Kushi LH, Weltzien E et al. Alcohol consumption and breast cancer recurrence and survival among women with early-stage breast cancer: the life after cancer epidemiology study. J Clin Oncol 2010; 28(29): 4410.

Hot flashes

21. Lyman GH, Greenleee H, Bohike K et al. Integrative therapies during and after breast cancer treatment: ASCO endorsement of the SIO clinical practice guideline. J Clin Oncol 2018; 36(25):2647.
22. Paddock, Catharine. Acupunture reduces hot flashes, night sweats in menopause. Medical News oday. MediLexicon, Intl., 25 May 2016. Web.

Fertility; pregnancy after breast cancer

23. Iqbal J, Amir E, Rochon PA et al. Association of the timing of pregnancy with survival in women with breast cancer. JAMA Oncol 2017;3(5):659.
24. Valachis A, Tsali L, Pesce LL et al. Safety of pregnancy after primary breast carcinoma in young women: a meta-analysis to overcome bias of healthy mother effect studies. Obstet Gynecol Surv. 2010 Dec;65(12):786-93.
25. Letourneau J, Ebbel E, Katz P. Pretreatment fertility counseling and fertility preservation improve quality of life in reproductive age women with cancer. Cancer. 2012;118(6):1710-7.
26. Valachis A, Tsali L, Pesce LL, Polyzos NP. Safety of pregnancy after primary breast carcinoma in young women: a meta-analysis to overcome bias of healthy mother effect studies. Obstet Gynecol Surv 2010 Dec;65(12):786-93.

Made in the USA
Las Vegas, NV
02 March 2023

68396447R00138